Somatization Disorder

in the

Medical Setting

Somatization Disorder

in the

Medical Setting

G. Richard Smith, Jr., M.D.

Professor and Vice Chairman
Department of Psychiatry
University of Arkansas for Medical Sciences
Little Rock, Arkansas

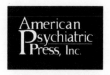

American Psychiatric Press, Inc.

Washington, DC
London, England

This report was developed under contract number 88-MO-305008-01D from the National Institute of Mental Health. Douglas B. Kamerow, M.D., served as the initial NIMH project officer, and Ann A. Hohmann, Ph.D., M.P.H., assumed that responsibility during the course of the study.

The opinions expressed herein are the views of the author and do not necessarily reflect the official position of the National Institute of Mental Health or any other part of the U.S. Department of Health and Human Services.

This monograph was previously published as DHHS Publication No. (ADM)89-1631.

American Psychiatric Press, Inc.
1400 K Street, N.W., Washington, DC 20005

Library of Congress Cataloging-in-Publication Data

Smith, G. Richard (George Richard), 1951-
    Somatization disorder in the medical setting / G. Richard Smith Jr.
    p. cm.
    Previously published : Rockville, Md. : U.S. Dept. of Health and Human Services, 1990.
    Includes bibliographical references and index.
    ISBN 0-88048-374-1
    1. Somatization disorder—Handbooks, manuals, etc. 2. Family medicine. I. Title.
RC552.S66S57 1991
616.85′25—dc20   91-6429
                                                                                              CIP

British Library Cataloguing in Publication Data

A CIP record is available from the British Library.

For SSS,

who is responsible for most of the good things.

Contents

Summaries

Foreword

People with somatization disorder are encountered frequently in primary care practices. A study by deGruy and colleagues (1987a) suggests that as many as 5 percent of those seen in primary practice settings may suffer from this mental disorder, which occurs as frequently as diabetes and urinary tract infections in these settings.

Despite its frequency, somatization disorder is often not recognized at all in primary care practice or is difficult to recognize as a mental disorder, since many of its somatic symptoms resemble those of a number of prevalent physical illnesses. Because of this underrecognition, many patients receive general medical care that is inappropriate and ineffective instead of the mental health treatment they require.

During the past decade, important research strides have been made in specifying empirically based diagnostic criteria for somatization disorder, elucidating the role of co-occurring psychiatric and substance abuse disorders, and developing effective treatments for this disorder. Effective approaches to treatment now include mental health counseling, the use of more specialized treatments such as group therapy to improve coping or socialization skills (Ford 1984), and the use of consultations by mental health specialists. All of these treatment approaches can help knowledgeable primary care physicians improve the course of this once-confusing and difficult-to-treat disorder.

Many primary care practitioners, especially those trained before these developments took place, have had little opportunity to stay abreast of the recent advances. Little of the available psychiatric research literature pertaining to the accurate recognition and effective treatment of somatization disorder has been translated into practical clinical advice for primary care physicians.

This volume was written to fill this knowledge gap by providing busy primary care practitioners with practical, state-of-the-art assessment, treatment, and management techniques for somatization disorder. It is intended to aid clinicians in more effectively recognizing and treating patients with this common mental disorder and in identifying when psychiatric consultation or referral is required. This publication includes up-to-date information on the history and epidemiology of somatization disorder, its comorbidity with medical, psychiatric, and substance use disorders, and the health care utilization patterns of patients with this disorder.

The volume's author, G. Richard Smith, M.D., has studied somatization disorder, its presentation in primary care settings, and its management. Publications from his research have appeared in many clinical fields, including psychiatry, internal medicine, family practice, and obstetrics-gynecology.

Using helpful illustrative case histories, Dr. Smith clearly discusses the challenge of diagnosing somatization disorder, the medical and psychiatric illnesses associated with it, the problems raised by neglecting to recognize it, and the bases for making the differential diagnosis. In addition, he suggests effective clinical means to treat and to manage primary care patients who suffer from this disorder. Finally, he offers guidelines on making a psychiatric referral.

For the National Institute of Mental Health, which sponsored the development of this volume, it represents an important aspect of our research mission: closing the gap between the findings of research and the clinician's office. Because primary care practitioners are a key resource in both recognizing and providing care for those with mental disorders, we are eager to ensure that clinically relevant results of mental health research, as found in this volume, reach clinicians quickly, in a form that will be accessible and applicable in their day-to-day practice. I believe that these goals are successfully met in this document.

Lewis L. Judd, M.D.

Acknowledgments

Numerous people have assisted with this book, and I would like to thank them for their help. I am concerned that some will be inadvertently left out, and I apologize for this in advance.

I am indebted to the numerous investigators and writers who labored so diligently to produce the research contained in this volume.

The origins of this monograph were within NIMH. The initial program officer was Douglas B. Kamerow, M.D., who began the process. Ann A. Hohman, Ph.D., inherited the project in its early stages and did a thoughtful and gentle job of overseeing it nearly to completion. David B. Larson, M.D., M.S.P.H., ably saw the project to conclusion.

Many independent reviewers gave most helpful comments on an earlier draft of this monograph. They are Drs. Charles V. Ford, Frederick G. Guggenheim, Ann A. Hohman, Kelly Kelleher, Peter R. Lichstien, Mack Lipkin, Jr., Z.J. Lipowski, Jack D. Maser, Gerald T. Perkoff, Stephen Snyder, James J. Strain, and Sarah Williams. While they provided much that was positive about the monograph, the mistakes and omissions are solely my responsibility.

Many of my research colleagues in Little Rock both supplied data and dealt with my unavailability during this process. They include Drs. Kathryn Rost, Jacqueline M. Golding, and T. Michael Kashner as well as Ms. Carla Baltz, Debbie Hodges, Dawn Neal, and Sue Randall.

The clerical work, including locating and keeping track of countless references, was cheerfully performed by Martha Mobbs, Kay Bradford, Joyce Massey, and Deloris Vest.

The editing and much of the drudgery was performed with skill and graciousness by Katherine Bullard. I am substantially indebted to her for her contribution. Sally A. Barrett undertook editorial management for the project for NIMH.

Major credit is due to my family, Susan Sims Smith and Roseann Claire Smith, who supported me during the ordeal of writing this book. They tolerated the long hours and the resultant lack of energy as well as lovingly welcoming me back into the relationships between drafts and when it was completed.

Introduction

The goal of this monograph is to provide primary care physicians and mental health consultants with current research findings on the recognition, diagnosis, and management of patients with somatization disorder. Somatization disorder is a recently described, chronic, relapsing psychiatric condition characterized by multiple unexplained somatic complaints.

It is not the intent of this monograph to present a thorough discussion of the process of somatization, which has been well described elsewhere,[1] but rather to directly address the relatively homogeneous group of patients diagnosed with somatization disorder. Management principles are also included for patients who do not specifically meet the diagnosis of somatization disorder but who appear to be diagnostically very similar.

How to Use This Book

Since primary care physicians and mental health consultants require different degrees of knowledge about this disorder, the monograph has been organized to be read at three different levels. The first level is as a quick reference guide to particular aspects of recognition, diagnosis, and management of these patients. In daily practice, a primary care physician can quickly pull this book from the shelf while the patient is in the office and obtain very specific, brief management suggestions to facilitate the care of the difficult patient. For example, when faced with the differential diagnosis between somatization disorder and hypochondriasis, the physician can look up "Differentiating Somatization Disorder" under "Diagnosis" in the contents, turn to the pages cited, and read the boxed summaries at the end of the appropriate sections.

The primary care physician who wants a quick overview of all aspects of somatization disorder can read only the boxed summaries at the end of each section plus the entire section on treatment. In this way, the entire field of somatization disorder can be covered in 20 to 30 minutes. The physician

---

[1]See, for example, Chodoff 1974; Ford 1983, 1984, 1987; Kaplan et al. 1988; Katon 1985; Katon et al. 1982, 1984a, b; Lipowski 1986, 1987a, b; Lloyd 1986; Merskey 1986; Smith 1985, 1988; Snyder and Pitts 1986; Westermeyer et al. 1989.

should probably read the material at least once in this manner to become generally familiar with it and subsequently use the monograph as a quick reference guide for management.

For the mental health consultant who works in a primary care setting and the interested primary care physician, this monograph provides (1) a thorough review of the research literature available on somatization disorder and (2) a topically directed annotated bibliography of the research literature. Consultants who need to be thoroughly grounded on somatization disorder, so they may serve as "experts" on these perplexing patients, should read the book in its entirety. The sections are designed to be neither inordinately laborious nor painful.

Terminology

The terminology in this field is confusing. Multiple terms are used to represent the same concept, while different concepts are referred to by the same name. Further, relatively subtle differences in terms (somatization vs. somatization disorder) have very specific meanings to those actively involved in the field, but at first glance, mean little to those not involved in the area. The following glossary is provided to help the reader understand better the material in this monograph.

BRIQUET'S SYNDROME: The eponym given to the disorder now called somatization disorder. It was initially proposed to avoid confusion associated with the term hysteria.

CHRONIC HYSTERIA: A term used in the past to describe the syndrome that eventually became referred to as somatization disorder.

CONVERSION: A psychological process whereby a physical symptom is substituted for an intrapsychic conflict or distress. This substitution often involves the temporary loss of physical functioning of a body part.

CONVERSION DISORDER: A psychiatric disorder characterized by conversion symptom(s).

CONVERSION SYMPTOM: A symptom, usually somatic, thought to be secondary to the process of conversion. Conversion symptoms are not pathognomonic of a particular disorder. Rather, they may occur in healthy people and as part of several disorders including somatization disorder and conversion disorder.

HYSTERIA: A centuries-old term replete with numerous meanings. For this reason, it is generally avoided except in historical discussions. This was the first name given to somatization disorder.

SOMATIZATION: A process whereby psychological distress is expressed in physical symptoms.

SOMATIZATION DISORDER: A chronic, relapsing psychiatric disorder characterized by at least 13 unexplained medical symptoms from a list of 37 criteria, with at least one such symptom occurring before the age of 30.

SOMATIZERS: Persons who have 6 to 12 unexplained medical symptoms in their lifetimes, with at least one such symptom occurring before the age of 30.

SOMATOFORM: A group of disorders with somatic symptoms that suggest a physical disorder, but for which no organic etiology can be demonstrated. There is presumptive evidence of a psychological basis for the disorder. These disorders are listed in DSM-III (APA 1980) and DSM-III-R (APA 1987).

Chapter 1

Who Are These Patients?

Somatization disorder patients as a group are well known to most primary care physicians. To further aid the reader in identifying who these patients are, three brief case examples are presented.

> Mrs. A. is a 47-year-old white female who presents to your office 2 weeks after she was eligible to see you under the new preferred provider plan that has just become available at the steel mill where her husband is employed as a laborer. She states that she has chosen you to be her primary care physician because of your reputation as a "thorough" physician in the community and because she has become quite disenchanted with many of the "careless" physicians in the community.
>
> Today she complains of chest pain and bloating that has bothered her for the past 6 months. Her chest pain is constant throughout the day. It keeps her from doing many of her usual activities, such as housecleaning; however, it does not keep her from bowling in her league. She describes her pain as sharp in quality and at times accompanied by a throbbing sensation.
>
> On your new patient information sheet, she has indicated that she is bothered frequently or occasionally by 42 of the 67 possible symptoms of your review of systems. Under history of family medical problems, she writes that she is the last child of six children, and that she has been sickly since birth.
>
> She reports that she has had eight operations. These included a cholecystectomy, an exploratory laparotomy where adhesions were found, a breast biopsy, a total abdominal hysterectomy at age 26 for pain and fibroids, a hemorrhoidectomy, and three D & Cs, one of which followed a miscarriage during which, she reports, she almost bled to death.
>
> She takes four medications on a daily basis—one for low energy, quinine tablets for leg cramps, a nonsteroidal antiinflammatory agent for her arthritis, and diazepam for her nerves. She notes parentheti-

cally that she has just run out of her diazepam and will need a new prescription from you.

Given all of the above, her physical examination is unremarkable except for mild obesity and appropriate abdominal scars for her listed procedures. Her resting electrocardiogram is normal.

Readers should note their subjective responses to this case. Usually, primary care physicians will wish that they had not been so fortunate as to have been considered "thorough" but can also usually resist the impulse to refer Mrs. A. to another physician.

Ms. B. is a 34-year-old mother of three children who is married to an attorney who has a senior position in one of the State's regulatory agencies. She is referred by her cardiologist because he believes she needs a primary care physician more than his treatment. She has been cared for by three cardiologists for her mitral valve prolapse and currently takes a low dose of a beta blocker for this condition.

When she sees you, she states that she is looking forward to getting to know you. As an aside, she adds that the last primary care physician she saw was not sufficiently attentive and understanding, so she decided not to go back.

She has no real problems today other than her mitral valve prolapse and ringing in her ears, the latter of which she has been told by other physicians is because of her excessive use of aspirin to treat her headaches. While it is also time for her every-3-months breast exam (an exam recommended to her by a previous physician because of her fibrocystic disease), the main reason she has scheduled this visit is to develop a relationship with you so that when she does become sick, you will be able to help her.

While Ms. B. does not work outside the home, she states that caring for three children is plenty of work. She is active in various community affairs including working in a literacy program.

Her past history reveals three Cesarean sections, two breast biopsies, and a cardiac catheterization. She states she was admitted to the hospital on two occasions for evaluation of her chest pain, one of which required the catheterization.

Ms. B. also states that she has had quite a few medical problems since early childhood—more, in fact, than most people her age. These problems began at age 7 when she was hospitalized for the evaluation of urinary retention. Ms. B. states that "they never could figure out what caused that."

She is dressed attractively in a red, tight-fitting silk dress that is stylishly short in length. She wears white hose and matching red shoes with 4-inch heels. She has three rings on one hand, two on another, and four gold bracelets on one wrist.

Her physical examination is within normal limits. She does have some mild nodularity in her breasts that appears to be fibrocystic disease.

From this presentation, you might expect that the primary care physician would initially feel flattered that an esteemed colleague had referred a prominent citizen to you for care. On the other hand, the astute physician might also wonder what lies ahead in the long-term management of this patient, especially considering the relatively extensive health care this woman has received for her age and her somewhat flamboyant clothing.

Ms. C. is a 48-year-old white female who is referred to your practice by a neurologist. She states that she has been completely disabled by her medical condition. Previously, she had been employed as a masseuse.

Ms. C. goes on to say that her neurologist, whom she had been seeing for shoulder pain, neck pain, and dizziness, had recently conceded that she "had too many medical problems" to be seen only by a neurologist and had, therefore, referred her to you. In addition to shoulder pain, neck pain, and dizziness, Ms. C. also complains of bloating and diarrhea, which have been intermittent for the last 3 months.

Ms. C. has had seven operations, including chest surgery when she was 6 months old; an appendectomy 18 years ago; two carpel tunnel releases; a hysterectomy; a gastric bypass; and a procedure for a perirectal abscess. She has been hospitalized both at the local teaching hospital and at another private hospital.

Ms. C.'s citing of the physicians with whom she has consulted is equally impressive. In the last 2 years, she has seen four physicians in a local multispecialty group, a primary care physician in a nearby city, and another neurologist.

On examination she is an obese white female wearing a black top, black slacks, and bright pink terry house shoes. Her hair is in rollers with a scarf covering the rollers. She tells you that she is just "too sick" to dress for the appointment.

She is extremely slow moving to and from the examining room and appears to be overtly cooperative but covertly resistant. Her speech is tangential, diffuse, and at times, rambling. She appears to be mildly depressed. Her physical examination reveals the scars of her surgery and, except for her obesity and moderate external hemorrhoids, is within normal limits.

At the end of the examination, Ms. C. states that she would like to sign a release of information so that you could forward copies of today's visit to her attorney who is assisting her in obtaining her disability income.

Ms. C. certainly has the capacity to develop into a difficult patient. Many physicians might feel inclined to schedule her next visit for 1 year later or simply suggest that she come back to see them only when she needs to. If either of these routes is taken, she is likely to be back in a week or two.

These three patients are all quite different. Two things, however, are common to each of these cases. First, the experienced primary care physician will probably intuitively sense that this person is going to be a difficult patient.

Second, each of these patients has somatization disorder, which is a chronic relapsing psychiatric condition characterized by the presentation of multiple unexplained somatic complaints. Fortunately, all three patients can probably be managed in a similar way—to the benefit of the patients and to the relief of the primary care physician.

Summary—Who Are These Patients?

Patients with somatization disorder are typically recognized intuitively by the primary care physician. Usually, physicians sense almost immediately that these patients will probably be difficult and briefly consider referring them to another physician. Once the patient is correctly diagnosed as having somatization disorder, a chronic relapsing psychiatric condition, appropriate management can be initiated for the patient's benefit and to the physician's relief.

Chapter 2

Historical Perspective

The history of somatization disorder is confusing. Essentially, two syndromes have been described over the centuries: monosymptomatic and poly-symptomatic. The monosymptomatic syndrome is currently recognized as conversion disorder, while the polysymptomatic syndrome has become known as somatization disorder. Historically, these two disorders have often been interrelated and commingled.

Early History of These Disorders

Somatization disorder has had many names and many antecedents. One such predecessor was the complex syndrome of hysteria, first recognized by the ancient Egyptians. The Kahun Papyrus, an Egyptian writing that dates from 1900 B.C., refers to many of the manifestations that today occur in patients with somatization disorder. An illustrative quote is a "woman aching in all her limbs with pain to the sockets of her eyes" (Veith 1977).

The Egyptians believed that hysteria was caused by upward dislocation of the uterus and displacement of other organs. The migration of the uterus throughout the body was the basis for the multiple symptoms developed by these patients.

Typically, they used one of two treatments for the wandering uterus. One treatment involved fumigating with precious and sweet-smelling substances to attempt to attract the uterus back to the womb. The alternative treatment involved inhaling or ingesting evil or foul-tasting substances to repel the uterus away from the upper part of the body where it had wandered.

The Greeks held fast to the Egyptian view of hysteria, as evidenced in some of Hippocrates' writings that mention the wandering uterus causing problems. The Greeks first used the term "hysterical" as an adjective to refer to a particular symptom. For example, they called the displacement of the uterus in the throat *globus hystericus*. Treatment for this symptom involved the application of foul-smelling substances around the neck, strongly perfumed wine in the mouth, and aromatic fumigations to the vagina.

The wandering uterus concept remained well in force throughout the Middle Ages and into the Renaissance, where writers continued to espouse the uterine etiology of hysteria. Richard Mead (1673–1754), probably one of the most successful English physicians of his time, stated that "no disease is so vexatious" as hysteria. He noted that it was common in maids, wives, and widows, and that ". . . while it may not be attended with great danger, it is frequently terrifying." For treatment, he recommended blood letting, applying cupping glasses to the groins and hips, inhaling fetid smells into the nostrils, and rubbing the thighs and legs (Veith 1977).

Doubts about the uterine origin of hysteria began in the 17th century with two prominent physicians, Charles Le Pois (Carlous Piso) and Thomas Sydenham, also famous for his discourses on gout and chorea. Sydenham not only dissociated hysteria from the uterus but associated it with the psychological disturbance known at that time as "antecedent sorrows," therein recognizing the emotional origin of the disorder. Further, Sydenham was the first to recognize the disorder in males. However, his important essay on the topic of hysteria was largely ignored.

Cotton Mather, a student of Sydenham and infamous for the Salem Witch Trials, wrote the first colonial medical text, *The Angel of Bethesda*. In it he, too, recognized hysteria, and as a loyal student of Sydenham, subscribed to a very similar formulation.

The French work on hysteria came not from private medical offices, as it had in England, but from large public institutions. Two public insane asylums, Le Bicêtre and La Salpêtrière, were the centers of this research. Philippe Pinel, best known for striking the chains of patients at the Salpêtrière in the true spirit of the French Revolution, placed hysteria under neurotic disorders in his disease classification published in 1813.

Pierre Briquet (1859) formulated a substantially different idea about hysteria. His report of the 430 cases he observed in the Hôpital de la Charité in Paris described a polysymptomatic disease. Unlike the prior emphasis on a single symptom, he emphasized the multisymptomatic patient with a protracted course. However, his treatise on hysteria, published in 1859, went largely unnoticed.

Briquet also recognized the disorder in men as had Sydenham before him. Briquet attributed the disorder to emotional causes and developed appropriate diagnostic criteria. His name was eventually attached to subsequent versions of the diagnosis because of the significance of his work.

Some time later at La Salpêtrière, Jean-Martin Charcot, a famous neurologist who also held a professorship at the University of Paris, devoted himself to the study of neurosis, hysteria, and hypnotism. Famous for his clinic where Freud observed the use of hypnosis in hysterical patients, Charcot emphasized single-symptom hysterical phenomena at the expense of the multisymptomatic patient. Like Briquet, Charcot, too, recognized the disorder in men, but because La Salpêtrière was for women, he worked exclusively with women.

Another French physician, Pierre Janet, recognized that hysteria was a general disease that affected the whole organism. He was a student of Charcot and presented many of his thoughts in his book, *The Mental States of Hystericals*, published in 1901.

Sigmund Freud is widely associated with hysteria. His early work with Josef Breuer led to two works—a preliminary communication on the practical mechanism of hysterical phenomenon, published in 1893, and one on his studies on hysteria, published in 1895.

Freud's discussion of Breuer's patient, Miss Anna O., was a landmark case that marked the beginning of the study of hysteria in psychoanalysis. Freud continued the movement away from the multisymptomatic patient and focused on monosymptomatic hysteria. He considered the psychic mechanisms involved in the development of hysteria as etiological. He eventually described a personality style or personality disorder that was associated with physical symptoms, but lacked the multisymptomatic focus.

Contemporary History of Hysteria

A landmark series of papers was published between 1951 and 1953 by Purtell, Robbins, and Cohen, who were later joined by Altmann and Reid (Purtell et al. 1951; Robins et al. 1952; Cohen et al. 1953; Robins and O'Neal 1953). These papers presented the first modern conceptualization of the multisymptomatic concept of hysteria.

They studied 50 patients with a diagnosis of hysteria using a systematic diagnostic process and reexamined them 4 or more months later (Purtell et al. 1951). They concluded that hysteria is a definable clinical syndrome with a characteristic clinical picture that begins before the age of 35. While noting the similarities of their work to Briquet's, they deviated somewhat from the latter's theories by suggesting that men did not have the disorder. Further, they reported a finding that has often gone unrecognized—that the prevalence of this multisymptomatic disorder in the general hospital is 2.2 percent of all admissions.

Followup work by Cohen et al. (1953) included a study of surgical procedures on 50 women with multisymptomatic hysteria. They noted the excessive number of operations—3.8 procedures compared to 1.9 procedures for the control group—and, by implication, the serious health care utilization problems of these patients.

The same group undertook an extensive search for men with somatization disorder in Boston area hospitals. Except for one case report that was published as an addendum, they found no cases of the multisymptomatic disorder in men that they had previously described in women. They concluded that somatization disorder is rare in men (Robins et al. 1952).

Published work in the modern era of hysteria ceased for a decade until two companion papers by Perley and Guze appeared. The first (Perley and Guze

1962) reported a followup study that confirmed the findings of Purtell et al. with respect to a definable clinical syndrome. It further demonstrated the diagnostic stability of the multisymptomatic concept of hysteria. Perley and Guze noted that patients had a 90-percent probability of meeting diagnostic criteria 6 to 8 years later. Their second paper (Guze and Perley 1963) reported that patients with multisymptomatic hysteria had a uniform clinical course that formed a chronic recognizable disorder with few, if any, remissions.

Guze went on to lead an extremely productive group of investigators who developed the contemporary diagnosis of multisymptomatic hysteria. The majority of these studies were conducted at Washington University in St. Louis.

Guze set the course for the development of research concerning hysteria by noting that the medical model is the sine qua non for progress in research and treatment of psychiatric conditions (Guze 1975). He argued that the medical model was built on diagnostic validity, which required a clear description of the disorder. This description could then be supported by demonstrating a common etiology or similar pathogenesis, which in psychiatry is always difficult. Two avenues could support diagnostic validity: (1) followup studies demonstrating a uniform course and (2) family studies demonstrating an increased prevalence in close relatives. These two particular types of studies were pursued with vigor over the ensuing 25 years. It should be stressed that while Guze had numerous collaborators on all of the aforementioned projects, he was the person primarily responsible for conceptualizing and validating multisymptomatic hysteria as we know it today.

The term "hysteria," with its ancient heritage, was further confused during and immediately after Freud's lifetime when the term took on new and more complex meanings that called into play various psychodynamic and psychoanalytic implications. For some, the term "hysteria" carried substantial pejorative connotations.

In 1970, Guze proposed that the eponym Briquet's syndrome or Briquet's disease be used to denote multisymptomatic hysteria. The disorder was known as Briquet's syndrome until the publication (APA 1980) of the *Diagnostic and Statistical Manual of Mental Disorders, Third Edition* (DSM-III). Ironically, after the decision was made to incorporate Briquet's syndrome as part of the new standard diagnostic nomenclature for American psychiatry, another separate, unrelated decision was made to drop all eponyms. Going back to the proverbial drawing board, a new name was created—somatization disorder.

In DSM-III, an attempt was made to simplify the diagnosis. Prior to that time, various diagnostic criteria had required 25 symptoms to be present, distributed over 10 symptom groups from a list of 60 possible symptoms— clearly, a cumbersome diagnostic schema (DeSouza and Othmer 1984). DSM-III streamlined the criteria to 14 positive lifetime symptoms in women (12 in men) from a list of 37 symptoms; moreover, the symptom group requirement was dropped. With the advent of DSM-III-R (APA 1987), the revised edition of DSM-III, the criteria were again modified, and the number of symptoms required for both men and women was changed to 13.

There are those who question whether somatization disorder is a single disorder. Some contend that the presence of other psychiatric disorders (psychiatric comorbidity) indicates a heterogeneous disorder (Liskow et al. 1986a). Others contend that there is a spectrum of disorders without clear demarcation between them (Ford 1983). While these arguments have merit, the currently available data argue for considering the disorder as a relatively discrete, homogeneous entity.

Summary—Historical Perspective

Somatization disorder evolved from an ancient concept of hysteria to psychodynamic concepts of hysterical phenomenon to, ultimately, a contemporary disorder characterized by multisystemic complaints. Many of the historical detours involved a monosymptomatic syndrome that is now known as conversion disorder. Somatization disorder has been known variously as hysteria, chronic hysteria, and Briquet's syndrome.

First recognized in the 19th century by a French physician, Pierre Briquet, contemporary work on the disorder began in the 1950s. Samuel B. Guze and his colleagues led a 25-year effort to characterize the disorder by providing careful clinical descriptions, documenting a uniform clinical course, and demonstrating the increased prevalence in first-degree relatives. The significance of this work was recognized by including the disorder in the DSM-III nomenclature, where it became known as somatization disorder.

Mechanisms

Psychosocial Mechanisms

Numerous theories abound concerning the psychosocial mechanisms involved in the process of somatization. By contrast, few theories have been proposed to account for the psychological basis of somatization disorder. Some people would argue that somatization disorder is simply the process of somatization carried to an extreme; they would submit that theories relevant to the process of somatization are relevant to somatization disorder.

Without entering into the debate, it is still appropriate to briefly discuss three areas relevant to this monograph: somatization as a social communication, as an emotional communication, and as a result of an intrapsychic dynamic.

Ford (1983, 1984; Ford and Long 1977) has discussed somatization as a social communication. Examples include the use of bodily symptoms to manipulate or control relationships—such as an adolescent girl's developing unexplained abdominal pain to prevent her parents from going away for the weekend. Similarly, somatization may be used to maintain relationships—as in the woman who receives nurturing from her husband only when she is ill. Other social uses of somatization include using it to gain disability or to divert attention. For example, a child develops or maintains a symptom to divert attention away from the conflict generated by the father's alcoholism.

Somatization may also be used to serve an emotional need or as an emotional communication. These, too, are well described by Ford (1983, 1984; Ford and Long 1977). Some patients may be unable to verbally express their emotions; therefore, they use symptoms to express their emotional state. Symptoms may also be used to symbolically communicate emotions, as they are in conversion disorders. Some patients use medical complaints as a coping device to deal with environmental stress. Finally, physical symptoms may be used as a solution to an intrapsychic conflict, again as in conversion symptoms.

Classical psychoanalytic theory has held that hysteria (conversion) represents a substitution of somatic symptoms for repressed instinctual impulses (Chodoff 1974). Freud postulated that the conflict was a phallic-oedipal one; however, more recent work has emphasized a pregenital conflict as well.

Pathophysiological Mechanisms

Some data are available on other explanations for somatization disorder. Neuropsychological testing by Flor-Henry et al. (1981) revealed equal bifrontal impairment of the cerebral hemispheres and nondominant hemispheric dysfunction in patients with somatization disorder. The authors suggested that dominant hemisphere dysfunction is fundamentally related to the disorder.

Abnormal psychological testing has also been noted in patients with somatization disorder (Liskow et al. 1986b). Compared to controls, these patients have significantly more scale elevations on the Minnesota Multiphasic Personality Inventory (MMPI). The authors suggest an MMPI screening scale for the disorder.

Preliminary evidence from Gordon and colleagues (1986a, b) indicated that patients with somatization disorder may have an abnormality in cortical functioning as evidenced by abnormal auditory-evoked potentials. In subsequent studies, the authors found that these patients responded more similarly than controls to both relevant and irrelevant stimuli. Hence, they had an impairment in attention (James et al. 1987, 1989). Other preliminary data indicate that somatization disorder patients may have electroencephalogram frequency abnormalities in the right frontal region (Drake et al. 1988). These data require much more extensive work.

Others have advocated that somatization disorder arises as a consequence of other disorders. Sheehan and Sheehan (1982) suggested that somatization disorder is a result of panic disorder. Orenstein (1989) proposed that somatization disorder is a sequela of a common diathesis that is shared by panic disorder and major depression. More data are needed to evaluate those proposals.

Genetic Mechanisms

Considerable evidence now demonstrates familial and/or genetic associations with somatization disorder. Patients with somatization disorder have been noted in several studies to have a higher than expected prevalence of antisocial personality disorder or, at the very least, manifest antisocial personality traits (Liskow et al. 1986*a*, *b*; Zoccolillo and Cloninger 1985; Lilienfeld et al. 1986; Guze et al. 1971; Cloninger and Guze 1970*b*). These data were derived primarily from patients seen in general psychiatric settings and in prisons. Some of the author's unpublished data appears to contradict these findings, possibly because our patients were not obtained from psychiatric settings but rather from primary care settings. In any event, the association with antisocial personality disorder occurs in only a relatively small percentage of cases in the general medical setting. Thus the association between somatization disorder and antisocial personality disorder is likely to be of only limited significance in the primary care setting.

Other work has shown that women with somatization disorder may selectively choose to mate with men with antisocial personality disorder (Woerner and Guze 1968; Cloninger and Guze 1975; Zoccolillo and Cloninger 1985). Here again, the association is only greater than random chance, not that a majority of patients with somatization disorder have spouses with antisocial personality disorder.

One interesting theory holds that antisocial personality disorder and somatization disorder may have a common genetic background, somatization disorder being the female expression of this genetic tendency and antisocial personality disorder being the male expression (Guze 1983; Lilienfeld et al. 1986; Cloninger et al. 1975). Work evaluating Swedish adoptees has shown that in the population, there are two types of somatization. One type, similar to somatization disorder, is associated with criminality in the biological parents (Cloninger et al. 1986*b*). While some evidence supports this theory, it remains theoretical.

Morrison (1983) indicated that patients with somatization disorder have a nonrandom birth order. This would indicate that factors other than genetics, e.g., the environment, play a substantial role in the disorder. A random birth order would be expected if a disorder were purely genetic. Accordingly, these findings would argue that somatization disorder is more the result of environmental rather than genetic influences.

Brown and Smith (1989) contradict this finding. We found a completely random birth order in 143 patients with somatization disorder. Therefore, at present, it is unclear which conclusion the reader should draw.

Summary—Mechanisms

Various psychological, social, pathophysiological, familial, and genetic mechanisms have been proposed to explain the origin of somatization disorder. At present, strong evidence supports an increased risk of somatization disorder in first-degree family relatives, indicating a familial or genetic effect.

Recent evidence pointing to the association of somatization disorder with antisocial personality disorder has also been accepted. At present, only limited data support psychological or social explanations for the disorder. However, women with somatization disorder appear to selectively mate with men with antisocial personality disorder and alcoholism.

Chapter 3

Prevalence

Mental Health Care in Primary Care Settings

As recently as 1986, findings from the Epidemiology Catchment Area (ECA) project conducted by the National Institute of Mental Health (NIMH) indicated that approximately one in every three Americans has or has had an acute psychiatric disorder in need of treatment (Robins et al. 1984). Further, 19 percent of Americans have a currently active psychiatric problem in need of treatment (Myers et al. 1984). When these somewhat surprising figures are combined with data on psychiatric manpower, it becomes very clear that speciality mental health services cannot possibly meet the service demand for these problems (Kamerow et al. 1986).

By implication, the major locus for psychiatric services is quite likely to be primary health care settings and, unless our organization of care changes drastically, such services will be provided by the primary care physician. This contention is further supported by empirical estimates that almost 60 percent of the care for mental illness episodes is provided by general medical providers (Schurman et al. 1985; Schulberg and Burns 1988).

Recent studies have also demonstrated that patients with psychiatric disorders are overrepresented in primary health care settings. Community-based estimates are in the 15- to 20-percent range for psychiatric disorders, while in ambulatory medical patients, the prevalence is 25–30 percent (Schulberg and Burns 1988). In patients with chronic medical conditions, Wells et al. (1988) reported a prevalence of psychiatric conditions in the 25- to 42-percent range.

Not only is the prevalence of psychiatric disorders in primary health care settings high, but these disorders frequently go unrecognized (Jencks 1985). Borus et al. (1988) found that practitioners in a health maintenance organization failed to recognize 66 percent of the psychiatric disorders present in their patients. This underrecognition can cause obvious problems since a patient cannot be properly treated until the correct diagnosis is made.

Recent advances in psychiatric treatment provide exceptionally effective means for treating many of the disorders seen in primary health care settings. For example, mood disorders can almost always be effectively treated, and prophylaxes can often be given as followup preventive measures. Significant advances in the effective treatment of panic disorder have also been made during the last decade (Katon 1989).

Unfortunately, the psychiatric care provided in primary care settings is at times inappropriate. As a result, patients are incorrectly diagnosed and treated, and primary care physicians become frustrated because their patients do not improve. For example, Callies and Popkin (1987) showed that antidepressant dosages for the treatment of mood disorders in primary care settings are insufficient and that the duration of the treatment is often inappropriate. Further, analgesics, antianxiety agents such as benzodiazepines, and similar psychotropic compounds are prescribed frequently in primary health care settings. While no clear evidence or statistics exists to indicate the exact magnitude of the problem, the prescribing of these drugs is undoubtedly excessive. Such factors work together to produce (1) patients who do not have the best outcome and are therefore likely to be dissatisfied with their health care and (2) physicians who desperately want good outcomes from their patients but often end up frustrated.

Summary—Mental Health Care in Primary Settings

One of the most common categories of disorders seen in general health care settings is psychiatric disorders, which affect approximately one in five Americans. Unfortunately, up to this time, numerous factors have impeded progress toward the successful treatment of these disorders.

Manpower in specialty mental health care settings is insufficient and will likely continue to be so, given the increasing demands for care for patients with these disorders. Further, the prevalence of psychiatric disorders is increasing in both primary care patients and patients with chronic medical conditions. Finally, health care costs for these individuals are great.

Other factors complicate the picture. Frequently, psychiatric disorders are unrecognized in general health care settings, so they remain untreated. Moreover, mental health care treatment in primary care settings has often proven inappropriate or inadequate given the current state of knowledge of psychiatric treatment efficacy. These factors underscore the tremendous importance of psychiatric knowledge among physicians in primary care settings.

Somatization Disorder

According to the ECA project, an estimated 0.13 percent of the general population, or one person in a 1,000, has somatization disorder (Swartz et al. 1990). One group of ECA investigators at Duke University used a somewhat different methodology and found the prevalence in the Piedmont region of North Carolina to be approximately 0.4 percent (Swartz et al. 1988). Estimates prior to the ECA study had been in the range of 0.4–2 percent of the population (Farley et al. 1968; Woodruff et al. 1971; Weissman et al. 1978). The ECA data probably underestimate the true prevalence of somatization disorder because of the limitations of the Diagnostic Interview Schedule (DIS), which was used for all the diagnoses in these studies.

Recent data indicate that the DIS may underdiagnose somatization disorder by as much as 31 percent compared to a careful clinical examination (author's unpublished data). This means that between 1 and 4–5 people per 1,000 in the community may meet the full diagnostic criteria for somatization disorder.

Other findings from the ECA project indicate that somatizers—people who have histories of multiple unexplained somatic symptoms but whose symptoms are not severe enough to meet diagnostic criteria—are relatively numerous in the population. Escobar and colleagues (1987*b*) estimated that 4.4 percent of the population studied at the Los Angeles site met an abridged construct of somatization. In Puerto Rico, Escobar et al. (1989) estimated that 18–20 percent met this abridged construct. Again, these estimates are likely to be affected by the systematic underestimation resulting from the DIS.

When somatizers are combined with somatization disorder patients, an appropriate estimate would be at least 5 percent, meaning 5 or more people per hundred in the general population may be somatizers. In fact, Swartz et al. (1990), who reported a subsyndromal form of somatization that they call somatization syndrome, estimated that 11.6 percent of the general population could be so classified.

While physicians in primary care settings see patients from the general population, they see a selected sample of the general population. This is evidenced by the number of patients with somatization disorder or multiple unexplained somatic complaints who present in primary care settings.

Since patients with somatization disorder believe themselves to be medically ill, one would assume they congregate in physicians' offices. Deighton and Nicol (1985) indicated that in a large group practice, 0.2 percent of the women between 16 and 25 years old possibly had somatization disorder.

DeGruy and colleagues (1987*a*) provided a much higher estimate. Their work indicated that as many as 5 percent of the patients seen in an academic family practice setting may have somatization disorder. If this is the case, then in a practice in which primary care physicians see 50 patients per day, 2 or 3 patients would probably have somatization disorder. Even if this estimate is high, the study clearly points out that patients with somatization disorder are overrepresented in primary care settings. Somatization disorder easily falls in the range of diseases such as diabetes mellitus and urinary tract infections in terms of the frequency with which it is seen in physicians' offices.

Early work by Woodruff (1967) and colleagues revealed that 1 in 50 women admitted to a medical ward had somatization disorder. DeGruy and colleagues (1987b) did similar work in the general hospital setting. They estimate that 9 of every 100 patients admitted to general medical/surgical services in the general hospital setting have somatization disorder. Another estimate based on their work placed the figure in the 3-percent range (Smith 1987). These figures indicate that somatization disorder is a major clinical entity in the general hospital setting.

Patients with somatization disorder are overrepresented among patients with certain disorders or with specific procedures. For example, 27 percent of women receiving non-cancer-related hysterectomies had somatization disorder (Martin et al. 1980). Two other studies reported an increased prevalence of 17 percent (Liss et al. 1973) and 28 percent (Young et al. 1976) in patients with irritable bowel syndrome. In another study, 13 percent of patients with polycystic ovary disease had somatization disorder (Orenstein and Raskind 1983; Orenstein et al. 1986), and 12 percent of chronic pain patients had somatization disorder (Reich et al. 1983). Folks et al. (1984) found that patients with conversion symptoms have a high probability (34 percent) of having somatization disorder.

Good data are not available concerning the prevalence of somatization disorder patients in subspecialty medical practices. However, anecdotal data and clinical wisdom indicate that somatization disorder patients are seen with substantial regularity in subspecialty practice. In a typical scenario, a patient with somatization disorder presents to the primary care physician with a new symptom. The primary care physician evaluates the symptom and believes that there is nothing medically wrong, overlooking the possible diagnosis of somatization disorder. In an effort to provide good care and not "miss" a diagnosis, he refers the patient to a subspecialist for an evaluation.

The onus is now on the subspecialist. A trusted colleague has referred a patient for an "expert" opinion. The subspecialist, wanting to be thorough and complete, performs various, often invasive, diagnostic tests. Indirect evidence from health care utilization patterns of somatization disorder patients indicates that this or some similar scenario must be operative since these patients undergo an excessive number of diagnostic procedures.

Presumably, medical specialists, particularly surgically oriented specialists, see somatization disorder patients quite frequently. Many of these patients undergo exploratory surgery or surgery for some type of symptom relief. The expected relief rarely occurs.

Given the number of symptoms that these patients will present during their lifetimes, there is a high probability of a chance association of some symptom and the presence of a false positive laboratory or diagnostic finding. For example, a 45-year-old man may be referred to a urologist for evaluation of dysuria. The patient may, in fact, have an enlarged prostate and when asked to describe symptoms, will describe characteristics of hesitancy and urgency. It appears to the urologist that a transurethral resection of the prostate is indicated. What was overlooked in this scenario was the fact that the dysuria was not a symptom of benign prostatic hypertrophy but rather a symptom of somatization disorder. It is, therefore, extremely important to identify patients with somatization disorder prior to surgery, because they frequently do not have the expected surgical outcome. Surgical, laboratory, and diagnostic procedures should be performed only when indicated by new signs of disease, not by symptoms (Monson and Smith 1983).

In psychiatric clinical settings, somatization disorder may be both underrepresented and unrecognized. Slavney and Teitelbaum (1985) found that 8 percent of patients with medically unexplained symptoms referred for psychiatric consultation had somatization disorder. Several small studies have estimated the prevalence of psychiatric patients with somatization disorder, but the rates varied widely (Saxena et al. 1988; Weller et al. 1983; Kroll et al. 1979).

The underrepresentation is likely due to the enormous resistance these patients have to understanding their disorder as a psychiatric problem rather than as a true medical illness. While these patients can eventually be referred and treated in psychiatric settings, the process requires skill, persistence, and time on the part of both the primary care physician and the psychiatrist.

Anecdotally, it appears that somatization disorder patients are underdiagnosed by psychiatrists to approximately the same degree that they are undiagnosed in general medical settings. Many psychiatrists do not even consider the diagnosis, so the diagnosis is rarely made.

Summary—Somatization Disorder

Patients with somatization disorder and those who have multiple unexplained symptoms but who do not meet criteria have only a modest prevalence in the general population. However, these patients congregate in general medical settings and in the general hospital.

> As many as 2 or 3 of every 50 patients seen in a primary care practice may have somatization disorder or near somatization disorder. These patients are almost uniformly unrecognized, undiagnosed, and consequently, mismanaged.
>
> Somatization disorder may be one of the more frequently seen disorders in primary care. Ironically, due to a *lack* of proper treatment and management, somatization disorder patients receive an inordinate amount of inappropriate care from specialists and subspecialists, which results in excessive diagnostic evaluations and surgical procedures.

Health Care Utilization

Changing physicians frequently or consulting new physicians—a phenomenon sometimes known as "doctor-hopping"—seems to be characteristic of patients with somatization disorder. While no definitive data exist on the number of physicians a patient with somatization disorder consults or the repetitiveness with which changes are made, these patients do see an inordinate number of physicians and change doctors quite frequently. This doctor-hopping confounds the management of somatization disorder patients since one of the prerequisites for successful management of the disorder appears to be a long-term relationship with one physician.

Excessive surgery was reported in patients with hysteria as early as 1953 by Cohen and associates. They found that patients with hysteria averaged 3.8 surgical procedures, while hospitalized ill control subjects had 1.9. Zoccolillo and Cloninger (1986a) compared surgical procedures in patients with somatization disorder and those with major depression and found that the somatization patients had three times more operations than the depressed patients. Morrison and Herbstein (1988) found that somatization disorder patients reported an average of 5.4 operations, while mood disorder patients reported 1.6 operations.

Lilienfeld and associates (1986) reported that somatization disorder patients had 4.3 surgical procedures per patient. Finally, in the author's unpublished study, patients with somatization disorder reported 5.2 surgical procedures with a range from 0–23. While no control subjects were evaluated for these latter two series, the general population is unlikely to have quite this many surgical procedures.

Frequently, patients and/or their physicians attribute these procedures to some particular indication, such as a patient who reports that she had an exploratory laparotomy for adhesions. However, rarely does a careful review of the physician's records show that any signs of obstruction were noted.

Whether the physician directly tells the patient or implies to the patient that adhesions are present or whether the patient infers it is unclear.

Whatever the case, patients with somatization disorder appear to have excessive surgery. It is fairly easy to understand how this can happen. Typically, the patient presents to a physician who is unaware of the patient's somatization disorder. The physician evaluates the symptom with diagnostic tests. The tests are normal. But the patient continues to complain, so the physician escalates the invasiveness of the diagnostic procedures. The symptoms continue unabated. In desperation, the physician may perform or refer for exploratory surgery to make a diagnosis.

Alternatively, in the dogged pursuit of organic pathology, physicians may discover abnormal, benign physical findings. If the physicians are not aware of the somatization disorder and only aware of the symptoms, they might mistakenly combine the symptom with the benign physical finding and believe that surgery is indicated.

An example of this phenomenon is a patient who complains of lower abdominal pain. If by chance she has tender, enlarged ovaries, the gynecologist may decide that surgery is indicated when typically, without the symptom of pain and only the finding of a slightly enlarged tender ovary on routine examination, no surgery would be performed. This type of surgery, of course, does not improve the symptom in the patient with somatization disorder. It may distract her for a period of time, but in most situations, the surgery is unnecessary and unhelpful and places the patient at increased risk of surgical complications. Such excessive surgery can be substantially reduced with appropriate management.

Because of the excessive number of operations and outpatient visits, patients with somatization disorder have extraordinary health care utilization. Data from the ECA project indicated that patients with somatization disorder as diagnosed by the DIS had 6.1 outpatient visits per 6-month period (Swartz et al. 1987). Ninety-five percent of these patients had seen health care providers in the previous 6 months versus 56 percent of the general population (Swartz et al. 1990). Of somatization disorder patients, 45 percent were hospitalized in the previous year compared to 12 percent of the general population (Swartz et al. 1990).

In addition to general medical service, patients with somatization disorder also use an abundance of psychiatric services. Seventeen percent of those in the ECA study were hospitalized on psychiatric services within the past year compared to only 0.5 percent of the general population; 56 percent were seen in psychiatric outpatient settings versus 7.5 percent of the general population in the previous 6 months (Swartz et al. 1990).

When hospitalized, these patients rarely receive the diagnosis of somatization disorder despite the high frequency of negative medical evaluations in somatization disorder patients (74 percent) compared to general hospital patients (21 percent) (deGruy et al. 1987*b*). In outpatient primary care settings, somatization disorder patients have been found to have 0.58 visits per month compared to 0.41 visits per month for outpatients without somatization disorder, and charges that were twice as much (deGruy et al. 1987*a*). Patients with somatization disorder have been shown to average 7.6 stays in the hospital per year and average 13.0 outpatient visits (Smith et al. 1986*a*, *b*). Smith et al. (1986*a*) found that the total health care charges for patients with somatization disorder in 1980 dollars were $4,700 per year or nine times the U.S. per capita personal health care expenditure.

Fewer data are available about the health care utilization of somatizers; however, some findings do exist from the ECA study. Men who somatize are more likely to use health care than men who do not somatize, while women who somatize are more likely to use general health care for mental health problems (Escobar et al. 1987*b*). Seventy-five percent of the patients who somatize have seen health care providers within the last 6 months compared to 56 percent of the general population, and 25 percent have been hospitalized in the last year versus 12 percent of the general population (Swartz et al. 1990).

Patients who somatize also use psychiatric outpatient services. Thirty-four percent were seen in outpatient settings during the last 6 months compared to 7.5 percent of the general population. They also require inpatient psychiatric hospitalization at the rate of 2 percent per year versus 0.5 percent of the general population (Swartz et al. 1990).

Summary—Health Care Utilization

Patients with somatization disorder have characteristic health care utilization patterns. There is frequent "doctor hopping" and excessive surgery. However, this excessive surgery can be reduced with appropriate management.

Almost half the somatization disorder patients are hospitalized in any given year. Their yearly health care utilization is nine times greater than the U.S. per capita health care expenditure. Much of this utilization may be unnecessary, especially since these patients rarely receive the diagnosis of somatization disorder.

Chapter 4

Course of the Disorder

Gender and Age

Somatization disorder was originally described in women (Purtell et al. 1951) and early reports stated that it was found exclusively in women (Robins et al. 1952). However, it is now recognized that somatization disorder does afflict men, but it is much less common in men than in women (APA 1987; deGruy et al. 1987*b*; Cloninger et al. 1986*a*; Kaminsky and Slavney 1976; De Figueiredo et al. 1980; Rounsaville et al. 1979; Smith 1987; Oxman and Barrett 1985; Maany 1981; Pittman and Moffett 1981). Guze (1983) stated that fewer than 5 percent of the somatization disorder patients seen by his group are men. Data from the ECA study indicated that the female/male ratio is 10 to 1 (Swartz et al. 1990). In a series of patients referred from primary care settings for a study of somatization disorder, the female to male ratio was 5 to 1 (Smith unpublished). Thus, it is important to at least consider the diagnosis of somatization disorder in men with multiple unexplained somatic complaints.

By definition, somatization disorder must begin prior to the age of 30. This does not mean that the patient must present prior to age 30. It simply means that the patient must have at least one unexplained somatic complaint prior to this age.

Data from the author's series of 126 patients with somatization disorder yielded an age range of 21 to 73 years with a mean age of 43 and a standard deviation of 11 years. In an attempt to find patients who met the criterion of 13 symptoms but with an age of onset later than 30 years, 151 patients with unexplained multiple somatic complaints were examined, and only two met this criterion.

The ECA data indicated that somatization disorder is just as prevalent among people under 45 years of age as among those over 45 (Swartz et al. 1990). Simply getting older does not affect the likelihood of having enough symptoms to qualify for the diagnosis.

The diagnosis is more difficult to make in a geriatric patient than in a younger patient. By definition, somatization disorder patients have a certain number of unexplained physical complaints. As the patient ages, it is increasingly difficult to attribute certain pain symptoms to a nonorganic origin. For example, if a 75-year-old female patient complains of joint pain, it is easier to attribute her affliction to some demonstrable joint pathology than it would be if she were 25 years old.

In the ECA study, the age of onset was under 10 years for 40 percent of the patients, and under 15 years for 55 percent. In women, the age of onset is usually at the time of menarche when they complain of dysmenorrhea and excessive bleeding (Swartz et al. 1990).

While there have been several small series on children with somatization disorder (Robins and O'Neal 1953; Livingston and Martin-Cannici 1985; Kriechman 1987), adolescents are more likely to have the disorder (Weller et al. 1983). By implication, the diagnosis of somatization disorder is rarely made before puberty.

There are now some indications that somatization disorder runs in families and that children of women with multiple unexplained complaints have children who also have multiple somatic complaints. Studies are currently under way to fully explain this relationship.

Coryell and Norten (1981) and Morrison (1989) noted that women with somatization disorder are more likely to be sexually abused as children compared to women with mood disorders. Morrison reported that 55 percent of the women with somatization disorder reported being molested as children while 16 percent of the mood disorder controls reported being molested.

Summary—Gender and Age

Somatization disorder is far more prevalent in women than in men. It does occur in men, however, and should be considered in the differential diagnosis of unexplained somatic complaints in men.

By definition, the first unexplained symptom must have occurred before the age of 30. The usual age of onset in women is at menarche. The diagnosis can be made at any age. Because of the development of other medical problems, the diagnosis is more difficult to make in a geriatric patient than in a younger patient.

Somatization disorder appears to run in families. Children of patients with the disorder may develop unexplained somatic complaints that represent the onset of the disorder. Usually, however, the children do not have enough positive symptoms to qualify for the diagnosis. Some evidence indicates that women with somatization disorder are likely to have been sexually molested as children.

Untreated Course of the Disorder

By definition, somatization disorder is a chronic relapsing condition. The etiology is unknown, and no cure for the disorder has been found. Proper management of this chronic condition is the treatment of choice. In its untreated course, the disorder usually begins in middle to late adolescence, but may start as late as the third decade.

Typically, patients develop a new symptom or symptoms during times of emotional distress. No data are available as to how long an episode of illness (relapse) lasts; it is the author's impression that a typical episode lasts 6 to 9 months. Quiescent periods (remission) may last 9 months to a year. However, it is unlikely that patients with somatization disorder will go more than a year without developing a new symptom or seeking some type of health care. As one indication of the course of the disorder, the ECA study showed that 95 percent of the patients with somatization disorder had visited a health care provider in the last 6 months (Swartz et al. 1988), while only 56 percent of the other community respondents had seen a provider during the same period.

Occasionally, patients in their 40s, 50s, or 60s become so frustrated with the physician's efforts to help them and with the medical profession in general, that they completely abandon visits to physicians. However, even during these times, patients probably remain symptomatic at a similar level of severity.

Periods of distress seem to coincide either with the onset of new symptoms or with increased health care–seeking behavior associated with some preexisting symptom. While no data exist on whether stress precipitates the relapse, there does seem to be an association.

This association is especially problematic since patients with somatization disorder are known for their chaotic social lives, often reflected in multiple divorces and remarriage, work disability, and marked interpersonal difficulties. Accordingly, they have an inordinate number of distressing situations. If many of these situations are associated with illness relapse, one can easily understand why relapses are so frequent.

In the author's series of patients with somatization disorder, 50 percent had been divorced at least once; those divorced had 1.4 divorces per patient. Several interesting reports have suggested that patients with somatization disorder engage in assortative mating (Woerner and Guze 1968; Cloninger and Guze 1975; Zoccolillo and Cloninger 1985), that is, they specifically choose a certain type of individual to marry and/or with whom to have children. Moreover, it appears that women with somatization disorder selectively choose alcoholics or men with antisocial personality disorder as their mates. This was confirmed in a recent study where primary care somatization disorder patients were interviewed about their husbands' alcohol consumption. The husbands were found to have a rate of alcoholism or alcohol abuse fourfold higher than the U.S. male population (Cook et al. unpublished).

As any physician who has treated patients with somatization disorder knows, these patients typically report poor health statuses. When standard measures for health status assessment are applied to patients with somatization disorder, these patients report that all aspects of their health—physical, social, and mental—as well as their general health perceptions are severely impaired.

When patients with chronic medical conditions such as hypertension, rheumatoid arthritis, chronic obstructive pulmonary disease, and insulin-dependent diabetes mellitus are compared to patients with somatization disorder, the somatization disorder patients report worse health than do those with chronic medical conditions (Smith et al. 1986a). In other words, patients with somatization disorder perceive themselves as "sicker than the sick."

This perception may be a helpful tool for primary care physicians to increase their index of suspicion for somatization disorder. When patients profess that they are substantially more ill than they actually are, somatization disorder should at least enter the differential diagnosis. Thus, while this concept is quite nonspecific, it may still serve as a useful clinical sign.

Further, since somatization disorder patients perceive themselves to be severely ill, it is not at all incongruous that they also usually deem themselves disabled from work. As evidence, Smith et al. (1986a) reported that 86 percent of the patients said they were disabled from work. With respect to full-time employment, three-fourths of the somatization disorder patients in the ECA study were not employed full time, compared to one-third of the patients without the diagnosis (Swartz et al. 1990).

Summary—Untreated Course of the Disorder

Somatization disorder is a chronic relapsing condition that usually begins in adolescence. There may be periods of relative quiescence or remission; however, these periods rarely last for more than a year, even in well-managed patients. The patients will still have symptoms. They simply may not consult a physician about these symptoms. Typically, patients develop new symptomatology during times of psychosocial distress. One way primary care physicians may increase their index of suspicion for making the diagnosis is that this type of patient reports being sicker than the chronically medically ill patient.

These patients often have disruptive social lives marked by interpersonal difficulties, difficulties that are further complicated by frequent episodes of anxiety and depression. Often, these patients seek time off from work because of perceived disability. To complicate matters, some evidence suggests that patients with somatization disorder select people to marry and/or to have children with who have a higher than chance likelihood of having antisocial personality disorder or alcoholism.

Psychiatric Comorbidity

Somatization disorder patients have much higher levels of depression than seen in the general population. In the somatization patients seen in psychiatric inpatient or outpatient settings, depression—including major depressive episodes—was manifest in 80–90 percent of the patients (Liskow et al. 1986*a*, *b*; Bibb and Guze 1972; Morrison and Herbstein 1988). These findings are amazingly consistent.

Patients with somatization disorder from primary care settings may be less likely to have depression; however, depression is still quite common in this group. In the author's current study, 92 percent acknowledged a history of depression. And yet, when these same patients were administered the DIS, only 40 percent had lifetime histories of a major depressive episode. An additional 9 percent had histories of dysthymia independent of a major depressive episode. Still, these lifetime prevalences are six times higher than would be expected in a general population (Robins et al. 1984).

Clinical wisdom indicates that patients with somatization disorder also have substantial problems with anxiety (Sheehan and Sheehan 1982). Cloninger and Guze (1970*a*) noted increased anxiety in female criminals with somatization disorder. Another study revealed that 28 of 41 patients with somatization disorder from primary care settings had a history of anxiety disorders (Smith et al. 1986*a*). Liskow et al. (1986*a*) reported on the systematic evaluation of 78 psychiatric outpatients who had somatization disorder. They found that 27 percent met criteria for obsessive-compulsive disorder, 39 percent had phobic disorders, and 45 percent met criteria for panic disorder. In the author's unpublished series, 34 percent of patients with somatization disorder had generalized anxiety disorder, 18 percent had obsessive-compulsive disorder, and 26 percent had panic disorder. In total, 66 percent had a diagnosable anxiety disorder (excluding simple and social phobias). These data provide support for most writers' clinical observations that patients with somatization disorder have substantial comorbidity with anxiety disorders.

Patients with somatization disorder may have an increased prevalence of alcoholism compared to the general population. In studies of psychiatric patients, 15–31 percent of somatization disorder patients had alcoholism (Liskow et al. 1986*a*, *b*; Bibb and Guze 1972; Martin et al. 1982). Sigvardsson et al. (1986) found that men with a somatization disorder–like illness had an increased prevalence of alcoholism. Several studies have noted that first-degree male relatives and husbands of patients with somatization disorder also have high rates of alcoholism (Woerner and Guze 1968; Arkonac and Guze 1963; Routh and Ernst 1984).

Of the author's subjects, 23 percent were noted to have a lifetime history of alcohol abuse and/or dependence; 1.6 percent of the subjects abused all other substances. This compares with approximately 16-percent prevalence of alcohol abuse and/or dependence seen in the general population. These data indicate an increased prevalence of alcohol problems but not of drug abuse.

Drug abuse, especially prescription drug abuse, has been deemed a complication of somatization disorder. Empirical evidence to support this is only moderate (Liskow et al. 1986a, b; Bibb and Guze 1972; Martin et al. 1982). The scenario used to explain prescription drug abuse is relatively easy to understand. Patients complain of a symptom. In an effort to relieve the symptom, the physician prescribes an analgesic, a hypnotic, or a tranquilizer. This medication improves the patients' symptom only moderately. They then present again. The physician either increases the dose or prescribes a more potent and possibly more abusable drug.

Personality disorders are longstanding patterns of maladaptive behavior that usually result in substantial interpersonal difficulties. Both histrionic personality traits and histrionic personality disorder are associated with somatization disorder (Lilienfeld et al. 1986; Kaminsky and Slavney 1983; Kimble et al. 1975). There is likewise an association of somatization disorder and antisocial personality disorder or antisocial behavior in men and women who are psychiatric patients or criminals (Liskow et al. 1986a, b; Guze 1964, 1983; Zoccolillo and Cloninger 1985; Cloninger and Guze 1970a, b; Lilienfeld et al. 1986; Guze et al. 1971; Spalt 1980; Guze et al. 1967).

In the author's study, 70 patients were administered the Structured Clinical Interview for DSM-III-R Personality Disorders (SCID II) (Spitzer et al. 1988). While no population norms are available for this instrument, 47 percent of the patients had evidence of at least one personality disorder. Specifically, 17 percent had histrionic personality disorder and only 4.3 percent had antisocial personality disorder. The most prevalent personality disorder in this group was avoidant personality disorder (28 percent) followed by paranoid personality disorder (24 percent).

Of note is that while 47 percent had one or more personality disorders diagnosed, 34 percent had two or more, 13 percent three or more, and 13 percent had four or more personality disorders diagnosed. Many of these subjects, therefore, can be considered to be severely disabled by their personality disorders, which are only diagnosed in the face of longstanding maladaptive patterns of behavior. The 26-percent prevalence of avoidant personality disorder may explain the severe social isolation apparent in somatization disorder patients.

Summary—Psychiatric Comorbidity

Most somatization disorder patients have severe problems with co-morbid psychiatric illnesses. Depression, the most common additional disorder, takes the form of major depressive episodes and dysthymic disorder. More than 90 percent of patients with somatization disorder acknowledge a history of depression.

Anxiety is also a comorbid condition frequently presented by the patient to the primary care physician. It may take the form of obsessive-compulsive disorder, phobic disorders, panic disorder, and/or generalized anxiety disorder.

Alcohol abuse/dependence is more frequent in somatization disorder patients than in the general population. Some studies have indicated that these patients also have an increased prevalence of drug abuse, especially prescription drugs. Recent studies of somatization disorder patients from primary care settings indicated an increased prevalence of alcohol abuse/dependence but not drug abuse.

One of the more disabling groups of comorbid conditions to plague somatization disorder patients is personality disorders. Almost half of all somatization disorder patients have at least one personality disorder.

Chapter 5

Diagnosis

DSM-III-R Criteria

Somatization disorder should be diagnosed according to the DSM-III-R criteria (Table 1). These criteria were published as part of DSM-III-R in 1987 and will serve at least until the issue of DSM-IV in the mid 1990s. The essential feature of the disorder is recurrent and multiple somatic complaints of several years' duration for which medical attention has been sought, but which apparently are not due to any physical disorder.

The diagnosis requires a lifetime history of 13 unexplained somatic symptoms from a list of 37 possible symptoms, the first of which must have developed before the age of 30. These symptoms must be of sufficient severity to require patients to consult a physician, take medicine, or change their lifestyle.

It is important to note that the physician need not be convinced that the symptom is real or has actually occurred. Patients' reports that they have the symptom are sufficient as long as the symptom meets the severity criteria.

Since the disorder frequently begins during adolescence or young adulthood, it is especially important to determine in women whether dysmenorrhea or excessive bleeding occurred around the time of menarche. This is a frequent time of onset for adolescent girls.

A patient can have somatization disorder even if a current or presenting symptom did not begin before the age of 30. A careful review of the earliest onset of any of the 37 symptoms for which the patient has had problems is necessary to make the diagnosis. While it may seem especially time-consuming and somewhat unnecessary for the busy clinician, it is well worth the investment because of the time saved in the long-term management of these patients.

Screening

It would help the physician in the clinical practice setting to have a tool for diagnosing somatization disorder, especially since the interviews required for such determination often take 45 minutes to an hour. Screening can be very

Table 1. Symptom list for somatization disorder

Gastrointestinal symptoms

1. Vomiting (other than during pregnancy)
2. Abdominal pain (other than when menstruating)
3. Nausea (other than motion sickness)
4. Bloating (gassy)
5. Diarrhea
6. Intolerance of (gets sick from) several different foods

Pain symptoms

7. Pain in extremities
8. Back pain
9. Joint pain
10. Pain during urination
11. Other pain (excluding headaches)

Cardiopulmonary symptoms

12. Shortness of breath when not exerting oneself
13. Palpitations
14. Chest pain
15. Dizziness

Conversion or pseudoneurologic symptoms

16. Amnesia
17. Difficulty swallowing
18. Loss of voice
19. Deafness
20. Double vision
21. Blurred vision
22. Blindness
23. Fainting or loss of consciousness
24. Seizure or convulsion
25. Trouble walking
26. Paralysis or muscle weakness
27. Urinary retention or difficulty urinating

Sexual symptoms for the major part of the person's life after opportunities for sexual activities

28. Burning sensation in sexual organs or rectum (other than during intercourse)
29. Sexual indifference
30. Pain during intercourse
31. Impotence

Table 1 (continued)

Female reproductive symptoms judged by the person to occur more frequently or severely than in most women

32. Painful menstruation
33. Irregular menstrual periods
34. Excessive menstrual bleeding
35. Vomiting throughout pregnancy

Source. Reprinted with permission from the *Diagnostic and Statistical Manual of Mental Disorders, Third Edition, Revised.* Copyright 1987 American Psychiatric Association.
Note. These 35 items represent 37 symptoms since numbers 26 and 27 are both listed as "or" for items that are not synonymous.

helpful to the physician simply because once the diagnosis is recognized, considerable management time is saved. In fact, deGruy (deGruy et al. 1987*a*), an advocate of screening who is himself a primary care physician, suggests that all primary care patients can be effectively screened for somatization disorder.

Several attempts have been made to develop screening indices for somatization disorder (Woodruff et al. 1973; Reveley et al. 1977). Currently, three published screening indices are in clinical use: one developed by Othmer and DeSouza (1985), another by Swartz et al. (1986), and finally, a modification of Othmer and DeSouza's screening index, published in DSM-III-R (APA 1987).

In one published comparison of these indices, a sample of 151 patients were studied who were referred from primary care settings because of multiple unexplained somatic complaints (Smith and Brown in press). The Othmer and DeSouza index resulted in a sensitivity of 83 percent and a specificity of 69 percent. The Swartz et al. and DSM-III-R indices performed in very similar fashion, with approximately 95-percent sensitivities and specificities in the 35- to 40-percent range. The DSM-III-R index is recommended since the Swartz index requires 5 positive symptoms from a list of 11 possible symptoms, whereas the DSM-III-R only requires 2 positive symptoms from a list of 7. All three indices are listed in Table 2.

If the DSM-III-R index is used, a positive screen in a patient with multiple unexplained somatic complaints indicates that the patient has a 69-percent chance of having somatization disorder (positive predictive value). Similarly, such a patient with a negative screen has an 81-percent chance of *not* having somatization disorder (negative predictive value) (Smith and Brown in press).

If patients have a positive screen, they require an evaluation for the disorder. This usually involves an extended return appointment with the primary care physician for assessment of all 37 symptoms from the criteria list. Psychiatric consultation may be sought to assist with making the diagnosis.

Table 2. Screening indices for somatization disorder currently in use

Othmer/DeSouza (1985)
  Threshold: 3/7
    Amnesia
    Burning in sex organs
    Dysmenorrhea
    Lump in throat
    Painful extremities
    Shortness of breath
    Vomiting

DSM-III-R (APA 1987)
(Othmer/DeSouza)
  Threshold: 2/7
    Amnesia
    Burning in sex organs
    Dysmenorrhea
    Lump in throat
    Painful extremities
    Shortness of breath
    Vomiting

Swartz et al. (1986)
  Threshold: 5/11
    Abdominal gas
    Abdominal pain
    Chest pain
    Diarrhea
    Dizziness
    Fainting spells
    Feels sickly
    Nausea
    Pain in extremities
    Vomiting
    Weakness

Summary—Diagnosis and Screening

Somatization disorder is diagnosed by the DSM-III-R criteria, which require 13 unexplained somatic symptoms from a list of 37 possible symptoms. These symptoms must have caused patients to (1) consult a physician, (2) take medicine, or (3) change their lifestyle. The first symptom must have begun before the age of 30, although the presentation and diagnosis can be made at any time.

The use of a screening index can be helpful to the physician because once the diagnosis is recognized, considerable management time is saved. In clinical practice, the most practical screening index is that published in DSM-III-R, which requires two positive symptoms from a list of seven to indicate a positive screen. If the screen is positive, then the patient has a 72-percent likelihood of having the disorder. The entire criteria list should then be administered or the patient referred for further evaluation.

Somatizers

Unless the reader is familiar with the work of Guze and his colleagues, it will seem quite arbitrary that a patient with 13 unexplained medical symptoms beginning before the age of 30 has somatization disorder while a patient with 12 unexplained somatic symptoms beginning before the age of 30 does not have somatization disorder. This has very practical applications in primary care since the patient who somatizes, that is, has 6–12 unexplained somatic complaints, is probably common in the primary care setting.

Guze and colleagues attempted to be quite rigorous in defining a disorder that has a uniform clinical course. Their work indicated that when the symptom number threshold is reduced, patients who have an atypical clinical course inappropriately receive the diagnosis.

As a problem in psychiatric nosology, the above information is quite interesting; however, for the busy practicing primary care physician, the issue is somewhat arcane or even irrelevant. In the primary care setting, the more pointed questions asked are "What is wrong with the patient with multiple but less than 13 unexplained complaints?" and "How should that person be managed?" The answers to those questions are simply not known. However, some research data, while indirectly relevant, provide some clinical wisdom that may be of help in management.

For the purpose of this discussion, patients with 6–12 unexplained medical complaints beginning before the age of 30 are defined as somatizers. Clinically, these patients present in nearly identical fashion to patients with somatization disorder. Like somatization disorder patients, somatizers focus much more on their symptoms than they do on any given disease. Similarly, they see multiple physicians and have had numerous surgical procedures, some of which are for questionable indications.

Data from the ECA researchers (Escobar et al. 1987a; Swartz et al. 1990) indicated that in a community-based sampling, those patients who somatize have increased health care–seeking behavior but are at an intermediate level between the general population and patients with somatization disorder. Community-based prevalence estimates are available for subsyndromal somatization, in this case defined as having between 4 and 12 unexplained somatic complaints. In all the ECA sites combined, 11.6 percent of the population had subsyndromal somatization (Swartz et al. 1990). While these data indirectly indicate that somatizers are similar to somatization disorder patients, the study is by no means conclusive nor does it prove that somatizers and somatization disorder patients have similar courses.

Through their clinical experiences, numerous writers have suggested managing somatizers with the same approach used with patients with somatization disorder. The implication is that these somatizers have a similar course and, therefore, may be managed in a similar way. No data are available concerning the course of somatizers. While specific management recommendations for somatizers are addressed in the following sections, it is important for the reader to understand that no empirical data are available to lend support to the above implied contention.

Summary—Somatizers

While important for nosological reasons, the criterion that a patient have a history of 13 unexplained somatic complaints is not particularly helpful in a busy primary care setting. Little is empirically known about patients who have 6–12 unexplained symptoms. Some data indicate that these patients have health care utilization similar to patients meeting diagnostic criteria. Clinical wisdom suggests that these patients be managed in a similar manner to those who clearly have somatization disorder.

Differentiating Somatization Disorder

An important aspect of successfully managing the patient with somatization disorder is making the correct diagnosis. Since numerous psychiatric and medical problems present with similar symptoms, careful attention to the differential diagnoses of these common syndromes is very important. Without proper diagnosis, proper management cannot be instituted.

Somatized Anxiety

A frequent problem seen in the primary care setting is somatized anxiety. This condition may result in psychic anxiety being transformed into muscle tension. For example, a new and somewhat insecure certified public accountant (CPA) may present to the physician's office complaining of the new onset of shoulder and neck pain. The CPA may have unconsciously converted his psychic anxiety to muscle tension in his neck and shoulders, thereby creating discomfort or pain. The same situation could be true if the CPA presented with a new onset of headaches. Similarly, the anxiety could produce abdominal pain with symptoms similar to irritable bowel syndrome.

Several aspects of the differential diagnosis are important to distinguish somatized anxiety from somatization disorder. Patients with somatized anxiety usually do not have a lifetime history of multiple unexplained somatic symptoms. Rather, they may have one or two symptoms that could have begun at any age. Second, somatized anxiety usually takes the form of musculoskeletal, sympathetic cardiovascular, or gastrointestinal symptoms. Usually, the patient has only two or three symptoms associated with the anxiety as opposed to the many symptoms manifested in the patient with somatization disorder.

Moreover, patients with somatized anxiety either have a chronic anxiety condition such as generalized anxiety disorder or have a situation in their life that produces the anxiety. This is not characteristic of a patient with somatization disorder, who may or may not have anxiety symptoms and who almost always is experiencing multiple distressing situations. Often, the patient with somatized anxiety has time-limited symptoms around the stressful life event. Finally, patients with somatized anxiety often have a symptom complex specific to that individual, such as the CPA who usually develops shoulder or neck pain during times of emotional distress or the high school student who develops crampy abdominal pain around examinations.

Somatized Depression

Depression is, unarguably, one of the most (if not *the* most) common psychiatric conditions seen in primary care settings. Typically, depressed patients present with persistently blue moods and some associated features of depression such as decreased appetite, decreased libido, insomnia, and loss of the ability to perceive pleasure.

Sometimes, however, depression may present as a somatized symptom. For example, a 62-year-old school teacher may present with diffuse mild abdominal pain that has lasted 4 to 6 weeks. She does not have a history of multiple unexplained somatic complaints, but she does have a sad facial expression and when initially questioned, acknowledges that she has difficulty experiencing pleasure. When questioned further, she admits that she has been increasingly despondent since her granddaughter moved to another state 6 months ago, adding that her granddaughter had been the center of her life while they lived in the same town.

Several points in this differential are important. The depressed patient usually does not have a lifelong history of multisystemic unexplained complaints. While numerous somatic symptoms may accompany depression, a history of unexplained somatic complaints beginning before the age of 30 suggests somatization disorder rather than depression per se.

Depression may often be episodic in that patients may have had similar symptoms at a previous time when they were depressed. When the patient over 50 presents with a new, obviously unexplained physical complaint, it is especially important to differentiate depression from the onset of a new somatic disease. In this situation, somatization disorder can be easily ruled out by simply taking a history of unexplained somatic complaints.

Panic Disorder

Panic disorder is another psychiatric condition that is seen with considerable regularity in primary care settings (Katon 1989). While some authors contend that the clinical picture of somatization disorder is often a sequela of panic disorder, only limited empirical evidence is available to support this contention (Sheehan and Sheehan 1982). Orenstein (1989) suggested a common substrate from which panic disorder, agoraphobia, major depression, and somatization disorder all develop. Further work in the area is necessary to adequately evaluate this contention.

Panic disorder is an anxiety condition in which patients develop very intense, acute episodes of anxiety lasting 3 to 5 minutes. These episodes are extremely uncomfortable and of such intensity that the patients often believe that they are dying or having a psychotic episode. This anxiety is accompanied by very characteristic somatic manifestations of anxiety, specifically tachycardia, palpitations, hyperventilation, and diaphoresis.

The differentiation from somatization disorder relies on the fact that these somatic symptoms of anxiety are expressly due to the panic disorder and its accompanying intense but short-lived anxiety. In contrast, somatization disorder is a chronic relapsing condition involving multiple systems with numerous complaints. Patients with panic disorder do not have a history of multisystemic unexplained problems.

Panic disorder may begin at any age whereas somatization disorder by definition always begins before the age of 30. Patients with panic disorder are more likely to present in the emergency room shortly after a panic attack. Rarely are they seen during a panic episode. On the other hand, patients with somatization disorder often have the symptom while they are being examined by the physician, and no associated anxiety or fear of a panic attack is evident.

Hypochondriasis

Hypochondriasis is a somatoform disorder whose essential feature is a preoccupation with the fear of having (or the belief that one has) a serious disease based on the person's interpretation of physical signs or sensations. Reviewed extensively by Barsky and Klerman (1983) as well as by Kellner (1987), hypochondriasis is essentially anxiety about having a particular disease or diseases. It is often thought of as psychic anxiety that is actually focused on normal somatic functioning, which is then interpreted as pathological.

Note that hypochondriacal patients present with concern that they have a particular disease, such as cancer. They may also have several symptoms. When asked if they are concerned about having a particular disease, they reply that they are very concerned. Their distress is not around a symptom but around the implication of the symptom, namely, a particular disease.

Patients with hypochondriasis may present over time with a series of worries. Nevertheless, this is noticeably different from the patient with somatization disorder who complains of various symptoms over time. Somatization disorder patients are almost indifferent to the possibility of their symptoms representing a diseased state. To reiterate, the patient with hypochondriasis is disease focused; the patient with somatization disorder is symptom focused. And, while hypochondriasis may begin at any time, somatization disorder typically begins in adolescence.

Conversion Disorder

Conversion disorder is a psychiatric syndrome characterized by the presence of a conversion symptom (Ford and Folks 1985). A conversion symptom is a loss of function, presumably based on an intrapsychic conflict. As an isolated symptom, the conversion symptom is probably prevalent in the general population. Conversion disorder is simply the diagnosis made when a conversion symptom is present.

Conversion symptoms may be a part of somatization disorder. Symptoms such as aphonia, paralysis, and blindness are conversion symptoms used to make the diagnosis of somatization disorder. In a series of patients with conversion symptoms in a general hospital, 34 percent had somatization disorder (Folks et al. 1984). However, somatization disorder differs from conversion disorder in that it is multisymptomatic and chronic beginning before the age of 30.

Numerous studies demonstrate that the clinical course of patients diagnosed as only having conversion disorder is extremely varied. In patients with multiple conversion symptoms, it is important to search diligently for the diagnosis of somatization disorder. If somatization disorder is correctly diagnosed, the clinician may have increased confidence that the patient will have a highly predictable course.

Somatoform Pain Disorder

Somatoform pain disorder is a psychiatric condition characterized by a preoccupation with pain in the absence of adequate physical findings that could account for the pain or its intensity. In this syndrome, previously known as psychogenic pain disorder, pain is the central focus, and psychological mechanisms are presumed to be of etiological significance or to contribute substantially to the patient's disability.

As with a conversion symptom, a somatoform pain such as chest pain may be a component of somatization disorder. However, the patient with somatization disorder has multiple symptoms. This assures the clinician of a much more uniform course than could be accounted for solely by the presence of somatoform pain disorder.

Factitious Disorders

Several disorders can be classified as factitious disorders whereby patients present with fabricated physical or psychological disorders. These disorders have been given various names such as Munchausen syndrome, Hospital Hobo, and so forth.

Patients who present with factitious disorders are thought to be malingerers, that is, they make conscious attempts to manipulate society for some overt gain. While Ford (1983) contends that patients with factitious disorder are quite similar to somatization disorder patients, to the author, factitious patients are quite different in that patients with somatization disorder do not make a conscious attempt to delude the physician. On the contrary, patients with somatization disorder genuinely believe they are medically ill. When the differential diagnosis of factitious disorder or malingering is considered, psychiatric consultants should almost always be considered to assist with the diagnosis, since the implications for the patient are substantial.

Medical Problems

Several medical conditions may initially be mistaken for somatization disorder because they are characterized by perplexing symptom complexes. These include multiple sclerosis, systemic lupus erythematosus, and sometimes, hyperparathyroidism.

Multiple sclerosis often presents with a perplexing picture of various neurological symptoms that are present for a while and then remit. Classical features of multiple sclerosis include impaired vision, nystagmus, dysarthria, intention tremor, ataxia, impaired position and vibratory sense, and bladder dysfunction. Most, if not all, of the above are signs of disease rather than symptoms—signs with which patients with multiple sclerosis present. Also, notably absent from the presentation of multiple sclerosis is the complaint of pain, which occurs frequently in somatization disorder patients.

Systemic lupus erythematosus (SLE) is another disease with a confusing presenting picture. Arthritis, arthralgias, fever, and central nervous system manifestations are common. SLE also has signs such as nephritis, pleurisy, pericarditis, anemia, leukopenia, and thrombocytopenia. These signs enable the physician to effectively differentiate it from somatization disorder. Further, SLE rarely presents with a loss of function, which may be one of the symptoms that appear in somatization disorder.

Hyperparathyroidism may present with nonspecific symptoms of the central nervous system, abnormal neuromuscular function, gastrointestinal symptoms, and pain in the joints and soft tissue. Hyperparathyroidism is, however, usually associated with recurrent kidney stones and/or signs of osteitis fibrosa as well as abnormalities in calcium metabolism.

Summary—Differentiating Somatization Disorder

The physician should be aware of three psychiatric problems that are frequently seen in primary settings and that may present as somatized symptoms—anxiety, depression, and panic disorder.

Anxiety typically presents as muscle tension, cardiovascular symptomatology, or gastrointestinal symptomatology and is almost always associated with overt signs of anxiety or stressful psychosocial situations in the patient's life. Depression usually presents with only a few symptoms and is often accompanied by other signs of depression such as blue mood, loss of the ability to experience pleasure, decreased appetite, decreased libido, or insomnia. Panic disorder is characterized by discrete episodes of intense anxiety and the associated concomitants of panic; somatic features are secondary. In any of these cases, somatization disorder would not be present without a longstanding history of multiple unexplained somatic complaints beginning before the age of 30.

Hypochondriasis can be differentiated because it is anxiety focused on a disease rather than on multiple symptoms. Factitious disorders and malingering also need to be differentiated. When these are suspected, they usually require a psychiatric consultant to assist in the definitive diagnosis.

A conversion symptom may be a part of somatization disorder; however, it is only one aspect. If only a conversion symptom is present, then the diagnosis is conversion disorder, not somatization disorder. Similarly, a somatoform pain symptom may be a component of somatization disorder. However, if this symptom is in isolation, or if the number of other symptoms is insufficient to make the diagnosis of somatization disorder, the patient will likely have a very different course.

Several medical conditions also need to be differentiated from somatization disorder. Disorders such as multiple sclerosis, systemic lupus erythematosus, and hyperparathyroidism may have confusing presentations; however, the clinician should look for *signs* of these diseases rather than relying on symptoms to differentiate them from somatization disorder.

Chapter 6

Treatment of Somatization Disorder in Primary Care

Once the correct diagnosis of somatization disorder is made, appropriate treatment can be implemented. Since the etiology of somatization disorder is unknown, and no treatment, either curative or ameliorative, has been found, it is probably more accurate to talk about the management of a patient with somatization disorder. Very few treatment or management studies exist for somatization disorder patients, but there is a broad general consensus concerning appropriate management strategies.[1]

Managing somatization disorder patients involves three levels of approach: (1) providing general management of a chronic condition, (2) conservatively treating certain symptoms for symptomatic relief, and (3) providing specialized care in specialized settings. Experimental data are available concerning management of the chronic condition, and some limited data exist on providing specialized care, but little or no research has been done on providing conservative treatment for symptomatic relief.

Managing the Chronic Condition

Management of the chronic condition known as somatization disorder has only been tested empirically in one study known to the author. Smith, Monson, and Ray (1986b) reported the results of a randomized, controlled crossover study of 41 patients with somatization disorder. This study tested the specific management recommendations detailed below. To date, the study has not been replicated, although a trial is currently under way.

Their findings revealed that when certain management strategies were

---

[1]Abbey and Lipowski 1987; Cloninger and Guze 1975; Cohen 1986; Ford 1984, 1986; Goodyer and Taylor 1985; Haberkern et al. 1985; Hyler and Sussman 1984; Katon 1985; Lichstein 1986; Lipowski 1986, 1988; Monson and Smith 1983; Morrison 1980; Murphy 1982; Oken 1984; Quality Assurance Project 1985; Ritvo and Thompson 1986; Smith 1985, 1988; Smith et al. 1986a; Woodruff et al. 1982; Zoccolillo and Cloninger 1986b.

undertaken by the primary care physician, the patients with somatization disorder maintained a constant health status. Simultaneously, their health care utilization decreased dramatically, and their satisfaction with their care improved over time.

The study's management approach includes (1) having the physician attempt to become the patient's main, and if possible, only physician; (2) setting up regularly scheduled outpatient visits at relatively frequent intervals (every 4–6 weeks); (3) conducting brief visits so that this management can fit into a busy primary care practice; and (4) during each visit, performing at least a partial physical exam of the organ system in which the patient has complaints.

Other important considerations in managing somatization disorder include understanding the symptom as an emotional communication rather than as the harbinger of new disease; looking for signs of disease instead of being symptom focused; and avoiding diagnostic tests, laboratory evaluation, and operative procedures unless clearly indicated. Finally, though this was not tested in the study, a goal of primary care management should be to get selected patients "referral ready" so that they are open to receiving care in the mental health sector.

The cornerstone for successful management of the somatization disorder patient is establishing a trusting relationship with the patient whereby one physician is the main and hopefully only physician that the patient sees. The constant "doctor-hopping" that frequently occurs in somatization disorder patients is countertherapeutic. In the author's experience, this typically occurs when the patient and physician are both frustrated with the unsuccessful management of the disorder.

Without a coordinated management approach, these patients do extremely poorly. Also, while it is possible to provide coordinated management with several physicians, it is much more cumbersome and probably much more work for primary care physicians than if they alone manage the patient.

Regularly scheduled visits are very important, especially in the first year of managing a new patient or in the period following an exacerbation of the disorder. In an effort to conserve health care resources and possibly avoid seeing difficult patients, physicians inadvertently contribute to their own management problems with these patients by telling them, "Nothing is wrong; come back and see me only if you need to."

This advice creates a situation whereby the patient must develop a new symptom to see the physician. Since seeing the physician is terribly important to the patient, physicians who attempt to manage patients with somatization disorder in this manner are likely to create many more problems for themselves than if they scheduled routine visits. By logical extension, primary care physicians who can capitalize on the patient's desire to see the physician actually expedite their management strategy for that patient.

The optimal interval between visits is unknown. The interval recommended in the study cited above was 4–6 weeks. Clinically, this seems to be appropriate. Once patients are stabilized, they may then look forward to the next visit and contain any new complaints until the next regularly scheduled appointment.

When establishing a new patient/physician relationship, during relapse, and during periods of psychosocial distress, 4–6 weeks is too long between visits. The interval needs to be shortened so the patient does not make extra visits or go to the emergency room.

On these patient-initiated visits, the patient usually presents new symptoms. New symptoms require more diagnostic effort and more of the physician's time. During periods of new symptomatology, intervals of 1 or 2 weeks may be required before patients begin to feel secure enough to stop initiating visits.

Once the patient-initiated visits stop, the primary care physician should not lengthen the interval for several weeks or possibly months. Then, the time may be gradually lengthened. Also, during the first year of management, it is generally not wise to lengthen the interval past 6 weeks, unless the patient suggests it.

When the patient presents with a new symptom, it is important to physically examine at least the organ system of which the patient complains. This examination serves two purposes: (1) it reassures the physician that no signs of organic disease are present and (2) patients receive real comfort from the examination. This examination may hearken back to the symbolic gesture of laying on of hands.

After obtaining a brief history of the symptom and physically examining the appropriate part of the body, physicians should then reassure their patients that they can find nothing seriously wrong, but that they are interested in both the patient and the symptom and want to follow the patient closely to make sure that the symptom resolves. This maneuver serves to reassure the patients and to teach them that the physician will provide ongoing care, doing what is necessary for the patients and their symptoms.

It is important that the physician communicate concern for the patient and the symptom. Further, it is best to avoid any suggestion that the symptom does not exist or that the symptom is not substantial. The patient actually hurts and does have the symptom. Suggestions to the contrary only serve to weaken the relationship and complicate the management.

The physician should understand that a new symptom is an emotional communication—that the patient is saying "I hurt" or "I am in distress." New symptoms presented by patients with somatization disorder are not the harbingers of new disease in the vast majority of cases.

Several authors suggest that when a symptom represents a new disease, the patient often presents in a qualitatively different manner, thereby cuing the physician to approach the problem differently. Since the physician is diligently examining the patient at each visit, looking for signs of disease, rarely, if ever, will an important new disease onset be missed.

Avoiding diagnostic procedures, laboratory tests, and surgical procedures unless clearly indicated serves three purposes. By deliberately refraining from using these procedures, the physician can (1) contain the health care utilization of patients who are extraordinary health care utilizers, (2) decrease the exposure to iatrogenic complications in patients who would normally receive an inordinate amount of procedures, and (3) decrease false positive laboratory tests in patients who have no real indication for the test.

The interpretations of laboratory and diagnostic procedures are based on set sensitivities and specificities (true positive and true negative rates) in patients who have appropriate indications for these tests. The criteria for a positive result established for patients with appropriate indications are not applicable to those without appropriate indications.

One possible resulting problem for clinicians is that they may be confronted with a patient who has a symptom (from somatization disorder) and a false positive laboratory test that appears to relate to the symptom but in actuality does not. This poses a very difficult management dilemma, usually forcing further diagnostic interventions, all of which will probably be for naught.

Most patients benefit from mental health care. With somatization disorder patients, this is much easier said than done. Willingness on the patient's part usually only grows out of a long-term patient/physician relationship—gradually and over time at that. Primary care physicians may, in a gentle, empathetic way, tell their patients that they understand the distress that the disorder must be causing. Physicians may then suggest that it might reduce the patients' distress to have someone who could spend more time with them than busy primary care physicians can.

In the author's experience, the above scenario works with a substantial number of patients with somatization disorder but should not be attempted before the physician/patient relationship is well established. It is very important that the patients not perceive that the primary care physician is abandoning them, but rather, that the physician still wants to follow the patient and will continue to be available as before.

Summary—Managing the Chronic Condition

The management approach to the patient with somatization disorder should take the form of brief, regularly scheduled visits so that the patient will not need to develop new symptoms in order to see the physician. The management checklist for treating a patient with somatization disorder includes: (1) establishing a strong patient/physician relationship where only one physician is providing care; (2) performing a physical examination of the area of the body related to the symptom of which the patient complains; (3) searching for signs of disease and understanding the symptom as an emotional communication rather than as a harbinger of new disease; (4) avoiding diagnostic tests and laboratory or surgical procedures unless clearly indicated; and (5) if possible, gradually moving the patient to a "referral ready" status to receive care in the mental health sector.

Conservative Treatment of Selected Symptoms

Several symptoms may need to be specifically treated in the somatization disorder patient. Typically, these are comorbid psychiatric and medical conditions. Since the patient needs a unified management approach, the proper management of these problems is important to the overall outcome of the patient. The specific problems addressed in this section are depression, anxiety, comorbid medical conditions, and disability.

Depression

Depression is the most common comorbid condition in somatization disorder patients. Depressed mood has long been recognized as an associated feature of somatization disorder. Depressed mood alone, however, is not an indication for psychotropic drug treatment since depressed mood in and of itself is not responsive to pharmacologic interventions.

Syndromes of depression, that is, constellations of signs and symptoms that together make up a discrete, clinical entity, should be treated in the somatization disorder patient. In the author's study of psychiatric comorbidity in somatization disorder patients, 9 percent were noted to have dysthymic disorder, and 40 percent had lifetime histories of major depressive episodes, "a depressed mood or loss of interest or pleasure in almost all activities for a period of 2 weeks" (APA 1987).

Regardless of the particular depressive disorder, the primary care physician should look for a persistently pervasive blue mood and the associated symptoms of depression—insomnia, anorexia, decreased libido, and anhedonia (the inability to experience pleasure). When this constellation of signs is present, aggressive psychopharmacologic management is indicated.

The drugs of choice for treating the depression syndrome are the tricyclic antidepressants. There are a wide variety of antidepressants to choose from; moreover, the clinician should remember to ensure that adequate doses are achieved for an adequate length of time and that the symptoms do resolve.

It is rare today for depression to be unsuccessfully treated. Therefore, if after aggressive management by the primary care physician the depressive syndrome does not resolve, the patient should be referred for psychiatric consultation and treatment.

Anxiety

The symptom of anxiety is very common among somatization disorder patients; many report chronic problems with anxiety. Much of this can be attributed to their inability to deal with the world and their poor social skills.

Treatments for anxiety vary depending upon the specific anxiety disorder. Both panic disorder and agoraphobia, a condition that at times can result from panic disorder, should be treated aggressively since combined pharmacologic and behavioral regimens provide superior results. The diagnosis and treatment of panic disorder are covered in a monograph by Katon (1989) in which specific treatment recommendations are provided.

Social and simple phobias are quite prevalent in the population (Kirmayer et al. 1988). In the author's unpublished series, they are even more prevalent in patients with somatization disorder. Unless the phobia hinders the patient in some substantial way, treatment is not usually indicated. When treatment is elected, the patient should be referred to a mental health professional.

Of all the anxiety disorders, the most difficult symptom that confronts the primary care physician, as well as the patient, is the chronic persistent anxiety as seen in generalized anxiety disorder. While the symptom of anxiety may be an associated feature of somatization disorder, usually the anxiety itself is severe enough to meet diagnostic criteria for generalized anxiety disorder.

For several reasons, this specific pairing of somatization disorder and anxiety can give rise to very problematic and difficult considerations in terms of primary care. The first difficulty is that only symptomatic treatment is available for generalized anxiety disorder. The benzodiazepines provide quite impressive symptomatic relief. Unfortunately, the very effectiveness of the benzodiazepines tends to undermine the treatment approach in the long-term management of patients with generalized anxiety disorder. As almost every primary care physician knows, because these drugs are so effective and because anxiety is so uncomfortable, patients often are reluctant to discontinue their medication.

Often, tolerance to the benzodiazepines develops, and the patient needs more and more medicine to achieve the desired effect. With a chronic lifelong condition, such dependency can obviously cause very serious problems. A new type of pharmacologic agent—buspirone—that is felt to be specific for generalized anxiety disorder and does not lead to tolerance or withdrawal symptoms, is now marketed in the United States. This drug has yet to stand the test of time. Hopefully, however, in several years the drug can be recommended as an appropriate treatment for anxiety associated with somatization disorder.

At present, the first line of treatment of generalized anxiety disorder in the somatization disorder patient is to encourage the patient to simply tolerate the symptoms. While encouraging tolerance or encouraging suffering of symptoms is not conscionable with the current direction of American medicine, few, if any, proven alternatives exist.

The next line of treatment is regular visits with an ample amount of emotional support. Emotional support can be surprisingly therapeutic.

Another possible line of treatment involves the use of biofeedback or some form of relaxation therapy such as systematic relaxation. Normally, these therapies need to be administered by a mental health professional. While their technologies are relatively straightforward, they are time-consuming and usually require special training.

As an absolute last resort, an extremely conservative, judicial use of antianxiety agents may be prescribed. As always with antianxiety agents, physicians should be relatively certain that they are the main physician that the patient is seeing. Prescriptions should be carefully monitored so that the dosage does not slowly increase over time. The patient should not be given multiple refills but should be required to return to the physician frequently for monitoring. And finally, by all means, the lowest possible dose should be used.

Comorbid Medical Conditions

Comorbid medical conditions also need to be treated and managed in the most conservative manner possible. In all cases, invasive diagnostic or therapeutic procedures should only be undertaken as a last resort, since these patients usually have poor outcomes.

The physician should be aware that patients with somatization disorder have what Barsky and Klerman (1983) described as amplified somatic styles. This means that they overrespond to almost any symptom. Therefore, the physician should exercise as much prudence as possible in the management of comorbid conditions, relying on frequent contact with the patient when the situation is serious.

Providing reassurance is extremely important when dealing with any patient who has a chronic condition. This is especially so in patients with somatization disorder.

The somatization disorder patient does not respond well to a complete description of all the various side effects of a medication. In this particular situation, it is much more important that the primary care physician tell the patient that the course of the condition will be relatively straightforward.

For example, in patients who develop moderate essential hypertension, a disease that can be easily controlled with medication, the physician should tell patients that the medication will control their blood pressure. It is unlikely that they will develop other symptoms or have other complications if the blood pressure is controlled. By having the physician check the blood pressure on a regular basis, both the physician and the patient are assured that the patient is doing well.

Disability

For most people, work provides structure for their lives, income for their families, and incentives for being healthy, the last of which many disability plans discourage. Unfortunately for patients with somatization disorder, disability from work is a very problematic issue. These patients are often quite incapacitated by their symptoms and often have a very limited capacity with which to deal with their world.

In one series of 43 patients with somatization disorder (Smith et al. 1986a), 86 percent said they were disabled from work. Zoccolillo and Cloninger (1986b) found that 26 percent had work disability compared to 4 percent of the control group. Considering the enormous societal costs that are incurred for disabled workers, work disability is a major complication of somatization disorder.

Just as work adds meaning and structure to healthy lives, work is equally important to patients with somatization disorder, and they should be encouraged strongly and repetitively to continue working. When that is no longer an option, the patient should be assisted in finding other, less distressing employment. Efforts in this direction could involve vocational counselors and probably rehabilitative services.

Rehabilitative services can be particularly helpful after a patient has been through numerous efforts to maintain employment. It is the author's usual practice to assist the patient in obtaining some form of disability payment.

Summary—Conservative Treatment of Selected Symptoms

The conservative treatment of selected symptoms in the patient with somatization disorder is important. Depressed or dysphoric mood should only be treated with psychotropic medication when a syndrome of depression is present. This usually means that in addition to prevailing depressed mood, the patient has insomnia, anhedonia, decreased libido, and/or decreased appetite. Usually, in any one of these cases, aggressive treatment with tricyclic antidepressants is indicated. The physician should ensure that the depressive symptom clears in an appropriate length of time after initiating treatment; if not, the patient should be referred for management by a psychiatrist.

Chronic anxiety in somatization disorder patients is much more difficult to treat. The physician should avoid prescribing psychotropic medicine but set up regular visits with the patient if possible. Biofeedback therapy or relaxation therapy is the treatment of choice.

The conservative, judicious prescribing of antianxiety agents should only be implemented if the primary care physician is reasonably certain that no other physician is also treating the patient. Regular followups with short intervals between visits is important if antianxiety agents are used. Likewise, the physician should treat comorbid medical problems conservatively, emphasizing reassurance and avoiding invasive proce-dures whenever possible since these patients typically do not have desir-able outcomes from such procedures.

Patients' efforts to obtain disability payments should be initially dis-couraged, with great effort directed to keeping the patients employed in their current occupation or one that is less demanding. Rehabilitation programs should be emphasized. If after considerable effort to maintain or regain employment the patient is still unable to work, it is probably best for the physician to support efforts at obtaining disability income.

Specialized Care

Group Treatment

Several authors have noted that group treatment for somatization disorder patients may be helpful.[2] Similar to suggestions for medical management, the authors are relatively uniform in their recommendations. Most suggest di-rected, time-limited group therapy where the emphasis is on ways to improve patients' socialization skills and ability to cope. Typically, these therapy groups are run by mental health professionals rather than physicians. While the solo primary care physician may lack a sufficient number of patients to form a group, moderately sized group practices probably have enough patients with somatization disorder or enough patients who somatize to form regular groups.

One moderately successful approach this author has used to encourage

---

[2]Ford 1984; Mally and Ogston 1964; Ford and Long 1977; Schoenberg and Senescu 1966; Schreter 1980; Valko 1976; Corbin et al. 1988. These reports, however, did not result from experimentally designed tests of group treatment. Corbin et al. (1988) did report a 33-percent reduction in office visits during the period of group treatment and the following 3 months.

patients to attend group meetings is to say that their purpose is to learn from one another ways in which they may better cope with their multiple medical problems. The physician should continue to see the patient on a regular basis, at least initially, and encourage the patient to continue in the group.

Advocating ongoing group psychotherapy is not likely to be a successful approach to treating the patient with somatization disorder, especially if the recommendation is offered early in the doctor/patient relationship. Patients usually become offended that the physician would suggest that their problem might be a psychiatric disorder instead of multiple medical problems. In addition, few somatization disorder patients are sufficiently psychologically minded for insight-oriented group therapy.

Other Specialized Treatment

The only other treatment approach mentioned in the literature is a trial of electrosleep in patients with somatization disorder. Electrosleep, now in disuse, is a form of central electrical stimulation at a subseizure threshold level. Scallet et al. (1976) found that specialized somatic therapies had no advantage over more traditional treatment approaches.

Summary—Specialized Care

Specialized care for patients with somatization disorder and those who somatize is likely to be limited to group treatment. Group treatment seems to be most effective when it is a time-limited, directive therapy focused on increasing the patients' socialization and coping skills.

Primary care physicians in group practice or multispecialty clinics probably have a sufficient number of patients with somatization disorder to offer at least intermittent groups. The physician's recommendation to attend group therapy seems to be most successfully received by the patient when it is offered as a way to help the patient cope with multiple medical problems. A direct suggestion or even inference that the problem may be due to psychiatric disturbance will likely meet resistance and be unsuccessful until a longstanding physician/patient relationship has been developed.

Indications for Consultation and/or Joint Care

Consultation with a mental health provider is often appropriate in making the initial diagnosis of somatization disorder. Since management of somatization disorder involves the long-term treatment of a chronic disorder, it is usually helpful to the primary physician to have another professional confirm the diagnosis. Such consultation tends to lower the physicians' anxiety about missing some esoteric diagnosis, thereby enabling them to more closely adhere to appropriate management guidelines.

Another indication for consultation or joint care is the presence of specific subspecialty problems. These fall into three categories: psychiatric, specific chronic conditions, and diagnostic questions.

Joint care with a psychiatrist or other mental health professional is important when other comorbid psychiatric conditions such as major depressive episode are present. Joint care facilitates an appropriate, prompt treatment of the comorbid condition, a condition that without fail adds to the disability of the somatization disorder patient.

When specific chronic conditions are present, the primary physician should care for the patient jointly with the subspecialist. In this situation, it is imperative that the primary care physician alert the subspecialist to the patient's somatization disorder and outline a conservative management plan with which the subspecialist should cooperate.

It is clearly unwise to ask subspecialist colleagues for consultation concerning a somatization disorder patient without alerting them to the patient's propensity for developing symptoms and complaining profusely about them. Unfortunately, the following scenario is more common than not: upon referral from the primary care physician, the somatization disorder patient sees a subspecialist. Unsuspecting and, what's worse, uninformed, the subspecialists unwittingly disrupt a carefully designed management approach because they believe that the referring primary care physician wants a symptom thoroughly evaluated and aggressively treated. As is usual with patients with somatization disorder, the symptom does not improve. The end result is increased health care utilization, a disrupted management plan, and a frustrated subspecialist.

Difficult diagnostic dilemmas can sometimes arise in patients with somatization disorder. In such a situation, the subspecialist who is assisting in the diagnostic evaluation should be alerted to the patient's somatization disorder and the need for a careful, conservative approach.

Specific indications should be present before diagnostic procedures are instituted. Again, abnormal physical signs rather than symptoms should be relied on to avoid unhelpful and possibly harmful procedures.

Summary—Indications for Consultation and/or Joint Care

Consideration should be given to having specialist or subspecialist consultation in at least four situations: when initially making the diagnosis of somatization disorder; when specific comorbid psychiatric conditions are present; when certain unusual comorbid medical conditions require management; and when difficult diagnostic dilemmas are apparent.

It helps to have consultation on the initial diagnosis since, once the diagnosis is made, the primary care physician embarks on a long-term management approach. Outside reassurance that the diagnosis is accurate would be helpful to the physician, given the commitment such a management approach requires.

If certain comorbid psychiatric conditions are present, such as a major depressive episode, the primary care physician may refer to a psychiatrist or other mental health professional to make sure that these comorbid conditions, which add to the patient's disability, are thoroughly and effectively treated. The management of certain comorbid medical conditions, especially those of an esoteric variety, often requires joint care with a subspecialist. It is very important for the primary care physician to alert the subspecialist to the presence of somatization disorder and to describe the specific management approach the primary care physician is taking.

In difficult diagnostic situations, subspecialist assistance may, again, need to be sought. And again, it is important for the subspecialist to know that the patient has somatization disorder and tends to overendorse symptoms. The subspecialist should be made aware that patients with somatization disorder have frequent untoward outcomes from diagnostic interventions and that signs of disease rather than symptoms of disease should be relied upon when making clinical decisions.

Indications for Referral

Many physicians believe that the simplest solution to the dilemma posed by somatization disorder is for that patient to go see another physician and never return to the primary care physician's office. This way of thinking is neither in the patient's nor probably in the primary care physician's best interest.

By contrast, it is usually in everyone's best interest for the primary care physician to make the appropriate diagnosis and embark on an effective long-term management plan for this difficult multisymptomatic patient. Two indications, however, when present, warrant referral.

The first indicates a physician's successful management of the patient with somatization disorder. After a long-term relationship has been established and the patient has been responding successfully to the management plan, the somatization disorder patient will likely be ready for referral to a psychiatrist or other mental health professional. In this situation, however, primary care physicians should still reassure the patient that they will continue to be available and will see the patient on a regular basis. Nevertheless, at this stage, the primary care physician can consider the management of the patient very successful, especially once the patient becomes successfully involved in treatment with the mental health professional.

A second indication for referral is when the negative feelings of the primary care physician toward the patient become so intense that it is no longer in the patient's best interest to continue receiving care from that particular physician. This situation occasionally occurs; when it does, the decision to refer should be made consciously rather than unconsciously.

The referral should be made in a direct manner. If at all possible, direct communication should occur between the referring physician and the accepting physician to make sure that continuity of care is maintained and that the patient is at least accepting of the referral.

Summary—Indications for Referral

Referral of a somatization disorder patient is most appropriate in two situations. The first instance is when the patient becomes "referral ready" and is able to accept direct treatment from a psychiatrist or other mental health professional. This usually occurs after a long, successful management course has been implemented by the primary care physician.

The second situation occurs when the primary care physician develops such negative feelings toward the patient that it is unwise to continue treating the patient. This type of referral should be directly discussed with the accepting physician so that continuity of care with the patient may be maintained, hopefully with a consistent management plan.

Chapter 7

Case Studies From Primary Care

These case studies are presented to assist the primary care physician in the recognition, diagnosis, and management of patients with somatization disorder. Case studies are used because medical education is often more enjoyable and effective when it is clinically based.

Several introductory comments are appropriate. The patients' clothes are described in more detail than is typical for medical audiences; the author and others have observed that many patients with somatization disorder dress noticeably differently from typical patients seeing their physician. While clothes are not generally pathognomonic, unusual dress may serve as a clinical sign for the physician to at least wonder about somatization disorder. Similarly, in several studies the patient's behavior is described since behavior, too, may be a clinical hint for the disorder.

Case #1

Ms. H. is a 38-year-old white female from a rural community 30 miles from the city. She has been married for 20 years to the same man who works for a public utility. She has an 11th grade education and is disabled from her work as a hairdresser.

She has been receiving her care from a publicly supported primary care clinic near her home. When her previous physician moved to another state, Dr. D., the new family practitioner assigned to her case, noted that her outpatient chart was 5 inches thick. However, the problem list did not include a single major chronic medical problem. She had reported 14 operations: a tubal ligation, five breast operations (four for fibrocystic disease and a fifth for reconstruction and breast implants), a cholecystectomy that included an appendectomy, a hysterectomy, bladder repair, an intestinal bypass, a stomach resection, and three D & Cs. During the past 2 years she received care not only from the clinic but also from a cardiologist, a psychiatrist, and a medical school teaching outpatient program. She was hospitalized at two different private general hospitals.

On her first visit to Dr. D., Ms. H. complained of shoulder pains. Since she was only scheduled for a 15-minute visit and the exam of her shoulder was within normal limits, Dr. D. rescheduled her for a more extensive return visit. On her second visit, for a followup of her shoulder pain, the pain was somewhat improved but still troublesome. Dr. D. administered the screening index for somatization disorder. She was positive for five of the seven symptoms. A third visit was scheduled in 2 weeks as an extended visit to obtain a careful history and physical examination.

On her third visit, she was noted to be positive for 20 of the 37 DSM-III-R symptoms with an age of onset of 12 years. On physical examination, she was noted to be an obese white female wearing a bright canary-yellow pants suit and black high-top tennis shoes. She also carried a 2-quart insulated pitcher of water with a straw, saying that her mouth frequently became dry. Except for her obesity and her abdominal scars, her physical examination was within normal limits.

During this third visit, Dr. D. said that he would like to have another physician see her, assisting him with making a correct diagnosis. She readily agreed and was seen on two occasions by a consulting psychiatrist who confirmed Dr. D.'s diagnosis of somatization disorder and made recommendations similar to those presented in this monograph.

On Dr. D.'s fourth visit with her, he began the management approach outlined herein, seeing her every 4 weeks. On her fifth visit to the clinic, Dr. D. noted that she continued to make emergency room visits once or twice monthly and called the clinic to come in for extra appointments about three times a month. At this point, he reduced the interval to every 2 weeks. Six weeks later, Dr. D. still noted too many emergency room visits and reduced the interval between her appointments to once a week. Over the next month there were no calls to the office and no emergency room visits. After 3 months of weekly office visits, the interval was extended to every 2 weeks—a change to which the patient readily agreed. She continued to save her complaints for her regularly scheduled visit and made no emergency room visits or calls to the office. After 3 months of every other week visits, Dr. D. increased the interval to every 4 weeks. This pattern was maintained for an additional 18 months with only two emergency room visits and an occasional call to the office.

At the end of this time, Ms. H.'s husband's employer changed their health insurance plan to a managed care plan. This required her to stop seeing Dr. D. and choose a physician from a panel of participating physicians. Even with Dr. D.'s and the consulting psychiatrist's help with phone calls and letters to arrange a physician who would be understanding of her problems, Ms. H. was unable to find a physician who would see her on a regular basis. Most indicated that they thought nothing was wrong with her and that she should only call them on an as-needed basis. About this time numerous emergency room visits began again as well as a plethora of telephone calls.

Comment: This case study illustrates that a high-quality patient/physician relationship is the backbone of successful management of these patients. When that relationship is disrupted for whatever reason, the patient's progress is likely to deteriorate, and the patient starts to backslide. This case also demonstrates how important it is to decrease the interval between regularly scheduled visits until the patient has no need to call the office for an extra appointment or go to the emergency room.

While at first glance this approach may appear to be an invitation to excessive use of medical care, it is by far the superior choice. The patient receives care on a regular basis, the physician can allocate time for a brief office visit, and the need for emergency room and urgent visits is dramatically reduced. All in all, the effectiveness of the care as well as its cost-effectiveness is substantially improved.

Case #2

Mrs. L.M. is a 54-year-old white female from a very rural area who was referred to a general internist in the city for evaluation of persistent back pain and multiple other complaints. The internist, Dr. S., hospitalized her. She noted that the patient was disabled from her job as a machine operator at a shoe factory. Mrs. M. gave a history of 10 operations: removal of a tumor from her right wrist, a D & C, a hysterectomy, three abdominal gastric operations, three breast biopsies, and leg surgery. She had received care from five different hospitals and seven different physicians in the last 2 years.

On physical examination, Mrs. M. was an obese, chronically ill-appearing woman who came to the hospital wearing her transcutaneous electrical nerve stimulation unit. She was cooperative and showed her various scars with a certain amount of enthusiasm. The remainder of her physical examination was within normal limits except for a decreased range of motion in the area of her lumbar spine and local muscle guarding with some tenderness in that area as well. Spine films did reveal some degeneration of vertebral bodies L2–L5.

Disallowing all back-related symptoms, Mrs. M. was positive for 16 somatization disorder symptoms with an age of onset of 26 years. Dr. S. made the diagnosis but asked for consultation with a psychiatrist to confirm the diagnosis.

Dr. S. discussed the management of Mrs. M. with the referring physician as well as providing him with reading material concerning the management of somatization disorder patients. Because of various circumstances, Dr. S. felt that the subsequent management by the referring physician was unlikely to go well. During the ensuing 12 months, Mrs. M. reported that she had been in bed 21 days, had made seven office visits to four physicians, and had been hospitalized for a total of 52 days.

Comment: Mrs. M.'s case illustrates that the diagnosis of somatization disorder can and should be made in the presence of comorbid medical conditions. Patients with somatization disorder do become ill, and their problems need to be appropriately diagnosed and treated. However, the management of somatization disorder should continue unchanged.

Case #3

Ms. A.P. is a 36-year-old white female who is a teacher in one of the local public school systems. She has been divorced but has been remarried now for a year. Her previous husband beat her, which she believes to be the origin of her problems. In addition, she was sexually abused as a child by her father. For the last 3 years, she has been seeing Dr. M., a general internist in private practice. Dr. M. had attempted to treat Ms. P. for depression with a tricyclic antidepressant without success because she stopped taking the medication because it caused a dry mouth.

Ms. P. was referred for psychiatric consultation and for management recommendations. When seen for consultation, she described three psychiatric admissions for depression. During one of the admissions, she was encouraged to return to school by one of the nurses. She entered psychotherapy and began to deal appropriately with the abuse dealt to her by her father and husband. She later divorced her husband and began making what she calls rapid progress. Since that time, she reports that her physical symptomatology has been substantially reduced.

She was positive for 13 DSM-III-R symptoms, with an age of onset of 10 years. She had a history of six operations: the removal of a cyst from the bladder, a hysterectomy, bilateral oophorectomy, a cesarean section, exploratory laparotomy, cholecystectomy, and a tonsillectomy as a child.

Her physical examination, as reported by Dr. M., was within normal limits. On mental status examination, she appeared to be a well-groomed white female looking her stated age. She was wearing a floral print jacket, navy skirt, cotton blouse with a large scarf, and moderately high heels. She was cooperative during the interview and fairly eager to be of help. She had some psychomotor slowing, her mood was blue, and her affect was appropriate to her mood. The remainder of her mental status examination was within normal limits.

By making a diagnosis of somatization disorder, Dr. M. was less likely to employ diagnostic procedures in the care of Ms. P. He was already seeing her on a relatively routine basis.

Comment: This case illustrates that depression is the most common comorbid psychiatric condition seen in patients with somatization disorder. At times, the depression is simply dysphoric mood; however, at other times, patients have major depressive episodes that require aggressive treatment. It further calls attention to the social chaos (abusive husband) that is common in many of these patients. Similarly, the history of childhood sexual abuse has also been reported to be prevalent in patients with somatization disorder.

Case #4

Mrs. V.H. is a 32-year-old white female who lives in a metropolitan area. She is a patient of the general medicine teaching service at a university hospital. She presented to the emergency room of the hospital complaining of a severe headache. She was evaluated in the emergency room, given pain medication, observed for 4 hours, and 2 days later, scheduled for an appointment to the group practice where she received her care.

In reviewing Mrs. H.'s record, Dr. W. noted an average of two emergency room visits per month for the last year. Within the last 2 years she had received care from two different emergency rooms, two different hospitals, a physician in another community, and another physician in a nearby suburb. She reported nine operations: a cholecystectomy, a D & C, three abortions, a tonsillectomy, two knee operations, and an appendectomy. When Dr. W. saw her, her headache had resolved, but she complained of chest pain that was sharp in nature, nonradiating, and not associated with exertion and that had been bothering her for about 4 months.

On physical examination, she was a casually groomed white female wearing a red and black sweater, blue jeans, and loafers and was carrying a bright yellow jacket. She had long blond hair. Her physical examination was within normal limits. On mental status examination, she was cooperative and pleasant, and her behavior was somewhat seductive. There was no pressure or eccentricities in her speech. She showed little hesitation in discussing intimate details of her life. Her mood was euthymic; her affect was appropriate to mood but possibly a little shallow. The remainder of her mental status examination was within normal limits.

She was scheduled 2 weeks later for a followup appointment. At this appointment she was positive for 13 DSM-III-R somatization symptoms. Her age of onset was 16. She was vague about the details of her life saying she was a part-time student and worked part-time as a singer. Dr. W. referred her for diagnostic confirmation.

When seen in consultation, it became apparent that her primary livelihood was as a prostitute. Further, she had a history of passing bad checks; there had been periods of her life when she did not have a place to live; and as an adult, she had been in physical fights. A substantial stress in her life was that at times she had so many somatic symptoms that she had difficulty working as a prostitute.

Comment: This case illustrates the association between somatization disorder and antisocial behavior and antisocial personality disorder. While this type of association is not present in the majority of somatization disorder patients, it is present in a higher proportion of the patients than would be expected by chance alone.

Case #5

Ms. D. was self-referred to an academic physician whose work with patients
with multiple somatic complaints had recently been publicized. A 43-year-old
white female, Ms. D. worked as a guidance counselor in a local high school.
She normally went to a primary care physician in private practice in her
community.

In her consultation with the academic physician, Ms. D. reported a history
of four operations: a hysterectomy, an exploratory laparotomy, and two thy-
roid surgeries. In the past 2 years, she had received health care from three
hospitals, two different otolaryngologists, and a general surgeon.

On mental status examination, Ms. D. was well groomed, wearing a grey
silk blouse, a grey skirt, and grey leather walking shoes. Her silver hair, which
was dramatically coiffured, gave her a strikingly matron-like appearance. Her
speech was somewhat tangential and circumstantial. Her behavior was cooperative, particularly since she handed the examiner a three-page, single-spaced
typed medical history that she had prepared on the morning of the consultation. Her mood was euthymic; her affect was appropriate to mood but somewhat schizoid and shallow. The remainder of her mental status was within
normal limits. Ms. D. was positive for 25 DSM-III-R symptoms with an age of
onset of 12.

Comment: This patient recognized herself as a patient with a somatization
disorder–like illness after having watched a 2-minute news story about the
author's work on a local TV news station. Her responsive action underscores
the fact that some patients with somatization disorder can evidence amazing
insight concerning their condition as long as the descriptions of the disorder in
the patient are not done in a pejorative manner. Particularly to be avoided are
phrases like "It's all in your head" and "I don't find anything wrong with you."

Case #6

Mr. N. is a 42-year-old white male who was referred by his primary care
physician for evaluation as part of a study of patients with multiple unexplained symptoms. An insurance underwriter, Mr. N. is married and has three
children. In the past several years, he has been through numerous evaluations
for inner ear difficulties. He has also had seven operations: tonsillectomy, eye
surgery, three ear operations, septoplasty, and the removal of a lipoma. In the
last 2 years, he was hospitalized on four occasions, one of which was a
psychiatric hospitalization. He has seen at least 10 different physicians in the
last 2 years.

On mental status examination, he was reluctantly cooperative and wore
sunglasses throughout the interview. When asked about the sunglasses, he
stated that they were his regular glasses and that he preferred tinted lenses. His

speech was not spontaneous and was circumstantial. He reported his mood as euthymic while his affect was constricted and moderately flattened. He was well oriented. He denied a history of hallucinations and ideas of reference. No delusions were apparent during the interview; however, his hospital records indicated paranoid delusions had been present. During the interview, his judgment was noted to be overly cautious and suspicious. His insight was limited.

When evaluated for somatization disorder, Mr. N. was positive for 16 DSM-III-R symptoms with an age of onset of 19 years. These 16 symptoms excluded any symptoms remotely related to his inner ear problem.

Comment: This case illustrates three points. The first is that men do have the disorder, and somatization should be considered in a differential diagnosis of men with unexplained somatic symptoms. Second, the diagnosis can be made in the presence of comorbid medical conditions. Finally, psychiatric comorbidity is probably higher in men with the disorder than in women.

Chapter 8

Clinical Scripts

Screening and Diagnostic Questions

DOCTOR: Ms. M., I would like to ask you some questions about some common symptoms you might have had at one time or another during your life. These symptoms do not have to be present currently but could have occurred at any time. For a symptom to be positive, it must have caused you to take medicine, see a doctor, or change your lifestyle. For example, if I asked you about headaches, and you had some, as most people have, but yours had not been severe enough to cause you to take medicine, see a doctor, or change your lifestyle, then your answer would be "no." Have you ever been bothered by chest pain?

PATIENT: Yes.

DOCTOR: Have you ever told a doctor about this?

PATIENT: Yes.

DOCTOR: What did the doctor say was causing your chest pain?

PATIENT: She did not know, she said it might be my nerves.

DOCTOR: When did you have this chest pain?

PATIENT: When I was in high school.

(This would constitute a positive symptom for somatization disorder.)

DOCTOR: Have you ever had shortness of breath?

PATIENT: Yes.

DOCTOR: Did you see a doctor about your shortness of breath?

PATIENT: Yes.

DOCTOR: What did the doctor say was causing your shortness of breath?

PATIENT: My asthma.

DOCTOR: Have you had shortness of breath at any other time except when you had asthma?

PATIENT: No.

(This would be a negative response.)

Discussion About Becoming the Patient's Main Physician

When initiating the management of patients with somatization disorder, it is important to become the patient's main physician to reduce that patient's propensity toward doctor-hopping. The discussion might go something like this:

> Ms. M., as we both know, you have a lot of symptoms and usually see a great number of doctors. I think it would be better for you to see only one physician as your main doctor. That way all of your care could be coordinated. You would then know that one person was attempting to understand your problems, and you would avoid the frustration of dealing with many doctors.
>
> I would like to be your main doctor. I believe we can work out a way to communicate so that you know I understand your problems, and you can feel assured that I am working with you in helping you feel better. Further, by following you closely, I can help evaluate any new symptoms you may develop to be sure that they do not represent something serious.

Referral for Mental Health Services

After the patient has been under your care for a prolonged period, a referral for mental health services may be appropriate. This should only occur after the relationship with you has been well established and the patient trusts you.

> Ms. N., I know that these numerous symptoms are distressing to you and that sometimes you must get discouraged by them. I wonder if it would be helpful for you to have someone to talk to about this distress—someone who has more time than I do and who may be better able to help you cope with these problems. This does not mean that I will stop seeing you. I will continue to see you just as before unless we both agree that it is not helpful—and if that becomes the case, I will still be available to you if you need me.
>
> If the patient refuses, you should offer to help her arrange it in the future if she would like.

Disability Request

Work is an important aspect of life. Patients with somatization disorder should be kept in the work force as long as possible. Frequently, the physician is approached to assist in obtaining disability payments. This should be discouraged as long as possible. One approach might be:

Ms. O., I understand that you are having difficulty working, especially with your many medical symptoms. While I know that to you it seems like things would be easier if you did not have to work, I think that is the wrong decision. In my experience, the longer you work, the better off you are. If your particular job is overly burdensome to you, perhaps you should consider changing jobs rather that obtaining disability.

References

Abbey, E., and Lipowski, N.J. Comprehensive management of persistent somatization: An innovative inpatient program. *Psychotherapy and Psychosomatics* 48:110–115, 1987.

American Psychiatric Association. *Diagnostic and Statistical Manual of Mental Disorders.* 3d ed. Washington, DC: the Association, 1980.

American Psychiatric Association. *Diagnostic and Statistical Manual of Mental Disorders.* 3d ed. revised. Washington, DC: the Association, 1987.

Arkonac, O., and Guze, S.B. A family study of hysteria. *New England Journal of Medicine* 268:239–242, 1963.

Barsky, A.J., and Klerman, G.L. Overview: Hypochondriasis, bodily complaints, and somatic styles. *American Journal of Psychiatry* 140:273–283, 1983.

Bibb, R.C., and Guze, S.B. Hysteria (Briquet's syndrome) in a psychiatric hospital: The significance of secondary depression. *American Journal of Psychiatry* 129:224–228, 1972.

Borus, J.F.; Howes, M.J.; Devins, N.P.; Rosenberg, R.; and Livingston, W.W. Primary health care providers' recognition and diagnosis of mental disorders in their patients. *General Hospital Psychiatry* 10:317–321, 1988.

Briquet, P. *Traite di l'Hysterie.* Paris: J.B. Bailliere et Fils, 1859.

Brown, F.W., and Smith, G.R., Jr. Birth order in DSM-III-R somatization disorder. *American Journal of Psychiatry* 146:1193–1196, 1989.

Callies, A.L., and Popkin, M.K. Antidepressant treatment of medical-surgical inpatients by nonpsychiatric physicians. *Archives of General Psychiatry* 44:157–160, 1987.

Chodoff, P. The diagnosis of hysteria: An overview. *American Journal of Psychiatry* 131:1073–1077, 1974.

Cloninger, C.R., and Guze, S.B. Psychiatric illness and female criminality: The role of sociopathy and hysteria in the antisocial woman. *American Journal of Psychiatry* 127:303–311, 1970a.

Cloninger, C.R., and Guze, S.B. Female criminals: Their personal, familial, and social backgrounds. *Archives of General Psychiatry* 23:554–558, 1970b.

Cloninger, C.R., and Guze, S.B. Hysteria and parental psychiatric illness. *Psychological Medicine* 5:27–31, 1975.

Cloninger, C.R.; Reich, T.; and Guze, S.B. The multifactorial model of disease transmission: III. Familial relationship between sociopathy and hysteria (Briquet's syndrome). *British Journal of Psychiatry* 127:23–32, 1975.

Cloninger, C.R.; Martin, R.L.; Guze, S.B.; and Clayton, P.J. A prospective follow-up and family study of somatization in men and women. *American Journal of Psychiatry* 143:873–878, 1986a.

Cloninger, C.R.; von Knorring, A.L.; Sigvardsson, S.; and Bohman, M. Symptom patterns and causes of somatization in men: II. Genetic and environmental independence from somatization in women. *Genetic Epidemiology* 3:171–185, 1986b.

Cohen, M.E.; Robins, E.; Purtell, J.J.; Altmann, M.W.; and Reid, D.E. Excessive surgery in hysteria—Study of surgical procedures in 50 women with hysteria and 190 controls. *JAMA* 151:977–986, 1953.

Cohen, S.I. Somatoform disorders—Symptoms and psychiatric implications. *Hospital Practice* 21(6):165–198, 1986.

Cook, K., and Smith, G.R., Jr. Assortative mating between patients with somatization disorder and those with alcoholism. In review.

Corbin, L.; Hanson, R.; Hopp, S.; and Whitley, A. Somatoform disorders—How to reduce overutilization of health care services. *Journal of Psychosocial Nursing and Mental Health Services* 26:31–34, 1988.

Coryell, W., and Norten, S.G. Briquet's syndrome (somatization disorder) and primary depression: Comparison of background and outcome. *Comprehensive Psychiatry* 22:249–256, 1981.

De Figueiredo, J.M.; Baiardi, J.J.; and Long, D.M. Briquet's syndrome in a man with chronic intractable pain. *Johns Hopkins Medical Journal* 147:102–106, 1980.

deGruy, F.; Columbia, L.; and Dickinson, P. Somatization disorder in a family practice. *Journal of Family Practice* 25:45–51, 1987a.

deGruy, F.; Crider, J.; Hashimi, D.K.; Dickinson, P.; Mullins, H.C.; and Troncale, J. Somatization disorder in a university hospital. *Journal of Family Practice* 25:579–584, 1987b.

Deighton, C.M., and Nicol, A.R. Abnormal illness behaviour in young women in a primary care setting: Is Briquet's syndrome a useful category? *Psychological Medicine* 15:515–520, 1985.

DeSouza, C., and Othmer, E. Somatization disorder and Briquet's syndrome: An assessment of their diagnostic concordance. *Archives of General Psychiatry* 41:334–336, 1984.

Drake, M.E.; Padamadan, H.; and Pakalnis, A. EEG frequency analysis in conversion and somatoform disorder. *Clinical Electroencephalography* 19:123–128, 1988.

Escobar, J.I.; Burham, A.; Karno, M.; Forsythe, A.; and Golding, J.M. Somatization in the community. *Archives of General Psychiatry* 44:713–718, 1987a.

Escobar, J.I.; Golding, J.M.; Hough, R.L.; Karno, M.; Burnam, M.A.; and Wells, K.B. Somatization in the community: Relationship to disability and use of services. *American Journal of Public Health* 77:837–840, 1987*b*.

Escobar, J.I.; Rubio-Stipec, M.; Canino, G.; and Karno, M. Somatic symptom index (SSI): A new and abridged somatization construct. *Journal of Nervous and Mental Disease* 177(3):140–146, 1989.

Farley, J.; Woodruff, R.A., Jr.; and Guze, S.B. The prevalence of hysteria and conversion symptoms. *British Journal of Psychiatry* 114:1121–1125, 1968.

Flor-Henry, P.; Fromm-Auch, D.; Tapper, M.; and Schopflocher, D. A neuropsychological study of the stable syndrome of hysteria. *Biological Psychiatry* 16:601–626, 1981.

Folks, D.G.; Ford, C.V.; and Regan, W.M. Conversion symptoms in a general hospital. *Psychosomatics* 25:285–291, 1984.

Ford, C.V. *The Somatizing Disorders.* New York: Elsevier, 1983.

Ford, C.V. Somatizing disorders. In: Roback, H.B., ed. *Helping Patients and Their Families Cope with Medical Problems.* San Francisco: Jossey-Bass, 1984. pp. 39–59.

Ford, C.V. The somatizing disorders. *Psychosomatics* 27:327–337, 1986.

Ford, C.V. Somatization. In: Soreff, S.M., and McNeil, G.N., eds. *Handbook of Psychiatric Differential Diagnosis.* Littleton, MA: PSG, 1987. pp. 195–235.

Ford, C.V., and Folks, D.G. Conversion disorders: An overview. *Psychosomatics* 26:371–378, 1985.

Ford, C.V., and Long, K.D. Group psychotherapy of somatizing patients. *Psychotherapy and Psychosomatics* 28:294–304, 1977.

Goodyer, I., and Taylor, D.C. Hysteria. *Archives of Disease in Childhood* 60:680–681, 1985.

Gordon, E.; Kraiuhin, C.; Kelly, P.; Meares, R.; and Howson, A. A neurophysiological study of somatization disorder. *Comprehensive Psychiatry* 27:295–301, 1986*a*.

Gordon, E.; Kraiuhin, C.; Meares, R.; and Howson, A. Auditory evoked response potentials in somatization disorder. *Journal of Psychiatric Research* 20:237–248, 1986*b*.

Guze, S.B. Conversion symptoms in criminals. *American Journal of Psychiatry* 121:580–583, 1964.

Guze, S.B. The role of follow-up studies: Their contribution to diagnostic classification as applied to hysteria. *Seminars in Psychiatry* 2:392–402, 1970.

Guze, S.B. The validity and significance of the clinical diagnosis of hysteria (Briquet's syndrome). *American Journal of Psychiatry* 132:138–141, 1975.

Guze, S.B. Studies in hysteria. *Canadian Journal of Psychiatry* 28:434–437, 1983.

Guze, S.B., and Perley, M.J. Observations on the natural history of hysteria. *American Journal of Psychiatry* 119:960–965, 1963.

Guze, S.B.; Wolfgram, E.D.; McKinney, J.K.; and Cantwell, D.P. Psychiatric illness in the families of convicted criminals: A study of 519 first-degree relatives. *Diseases of the Nervous System* 28:651–659, 1967.

Guze, S.B.; Woodruff, R.A., Jr.; and Clayton, P.J. Hysteria and antisocial behavior: Further evidence of an association. *American Journal of Psychiatry* 127:957–960, 1971.

Haberkern, R.; Schmitt, R.F.; and Taylor, C. Briquet's syndrome in adolescence. *Southern Medical Journal* 78:919–923, 1985.

Hyler, S.E., and Sussman, N. Somatoform disorders: Before and after DSM-III. *Hospital and Community Psychiatry* 35:469–478, 1984.

James, L.; Singer, A.; Zurnyski, Y.; Gordon, E.; Kraiuhin, C.J.; Harris, A.; Howson, A.J.; and Meares, R. Evoked response potentials and regional cerebral blood flow in somatization disorder. *Psychotherapy and Psychosomatics* 47:190–196, 1987.

James, L.; Gordon, E.; Kraiuhin, C.; and Meares, R. Selective attention and auditory event-related potentials in somatization disorder. *Comprehensive Psychiatry* 30:84–89, 1989.

Jencks, S.F. Recognition of mental distress and diagnosis of mental disorder in primary care. *JAMA* 253:1903–1907, 1985.

Kamerow, D.B.; Pincus, H.A.; and Macdonald, D.I. Alcohol abuse, other drug abuse, and mental disorders in medical practice. *JAMA* 255:2054–2057, 1986.

Kaminsky, M.J., and Slavney, P.R. Methodology and personality in Briquet's syndrome: A reappraisal. *American Journal of Psychiatry* 133:85–88, 1976.

Kaminsky, M.J., and Slavney, P.R. Hysterical and obsessional features in patients with Briquet's syndrome (somatization disorder). *Psychological Medicine* 13:111–120, 1983.

Kaplan, C.; Lipkin, M., Jr.; and Gordon, G.H. Somatization in primary care: Patients with unexplained and vexing medical complaints. *Journal of General Internal Medicine* 3:177–190, 1988.

Katon, W. Somatization in primary care. *Journal of Family Practice* 21:257–258, 1985.

Katon, W. *Panic Disorder in the Medical Setting.* National Institute of Mental Health, DHHS Pub. No. (ADM)89-1629. Washington, DC: Supt. of Docs., U.S. Govt. Print. Off., 1989.

Katon, W.; Kleinman, A.; and Rosen, G. Depression and somatization: A review. *American Journal of Medicine* 72:127–135, 1982.

Katon, W.; Ries, R.K.; and Kleinman, A. Part II: A prospective DSM-III study of 100 consecutive somatization patients. *Comprehensive Psychiatry* 25:305–314, 1984*a*.

Katon, W.; Ries, R.K.; and Kleinman, A. The prevalence of somatization in primary care. *Comprehensive Psychiatry* 25:208–215, 1984*b*.

Kellner, R. Hypochondriasis and somatization. *JAMA* 258:2718–2722, 1987.

Kimble, R.; Williams, J.G.; and Agras, S. A comparison of two methods of diagnosing hysteria. *American Journal of Psychiatry* 132:1197–1199, 1975.

Kirmayer, L.J.; Robbins, J.M.; and Kapusta, M.A. Somatization and depression in fibromyalgia syndrome. *American Journal of Psychiatry* 145:950–954, 1988.

Kriechman, A.M. Siblings with somatoform disorders in childhood and adolescence. *Journal of the American Academy of Child and Adolescent Psychiatry* 26:226–231, 1987.

Kroll, P.; Chamberlain, K.R.; and Halpern, J. The diagnosis of Briquet's syndrome in a male population. *Journal of Nervous and Mental Disease* 167:171–174, 1979.

Lichstein, P.R. Caring for the patient with multiple somatic complaints. *Southern Medical Journal* 79:310–314, 1986.

Lilienfeld, S.O.; Van Valkenburg, C.; Larntz, K.; and Akiskal, H.S. The relationship of histrionic personality disorder to antisocial personality and somatization disorders. *American Journal of Psychiatry* 143:718–722, 1986.

Lipowski, Z.J. Somatization: A borderland between medicine and psychiatry. *Canadian Medical Association Journal* 135:609–614, 1986.

Lipowski, Z.J. Somatization: Medicine's unsolved problem. *Psychosomatics* 28:294–297, 1987*a*.

Lipowski, Z.J. Somatization: The experience and communications of psychological distress as somatic symptoms. *Psychotherapy and Psychosomatics* 47:160–167, 1987*b*.

Lipowski, Z.J. An inpatient programme for persistent somatizers. *Canadian Journal of Psychiatry* 33:275–278, 1988.

Liskow, B.; Othmer, E.; Penick, E.C.; DeSouza, C.; and Gabrielli, W. Is Briquet's syndrome a heterogeneous disorder? *American Journal of Psychiatry* 143:626–629, 1986*a*.

Liskow, B.; Penick, E.C.; Powell, B.J.; Haefele, W.F.; and Campbell, J.L. Inpatients with Briquet's syndrome: Presence of additional psychiatric syndromes and MMPI results. *Comprehensive Psychiatry* 27:461–470, 1986*b*.

Liss, J.L.; Alpers, D.; and Woodruff, R.A., Jr. The irritable colon syndrome and psychiatric illness. *Diseases of the Nervous System* 34:151–157, 1973.

Livingston, R., and Martin-Cannici, C. Multiple somatic complaints and possible somatization disorder in prepubertal children. *Journal of the American Academy of Child Psychiatry* 24:603–607, 1985.

Lloyd, G.G. Review article—Psychiatric syndromes with a somatic presentation. *Journal of Psychosomatic Research* 30:113–120, 1986.

Maany, I. Treatment of depression associated with Briquet's syndrome. *American Journal of Psychiatry* 138:373–376, 1981.

Mally, M.A., and Ogston, W.D. Treatment of the "untreatables." *International Journal of Group Psychotherapy* 14:369–374, 1964.

Martin, R.L.; Roberts, W.V.; and Clayton, P.J. Psychiatric status after hysterectomy. *JAMA* 244:350–353, 1980.

Martin, R.L.; Cloninger, C.R.; and Guze, S.B. The natural history of somatization and substance abuse in women criminals: A six year follow-up. *Comprehensive Psychiatry* 23:528–536, 1982.

Merskey, H. The importance of hysteria. *British Journal of Psychiatry* 149:23–28, 1986.

Monson, R.A., and Smith, G.R., Jr. Current concepts in psychiatry: Somatization disorder in primary care. *New England Journal of Medicine* 308:1464–1465, 1983.

Morrison, J. Adult psychiatric disorders in parents of hyperactive children. *American Journal of Psychiatry* 137:825–827, 1980.

Morrison, J.R. Early birth order in Briquet's syndrome. *American Journal of Psychiatry* 140:1596–1598, 1983.

Morrison, J. Childhood sexual histories of women with somatization disorder. *American Journal of Psychiatry* 146:239–241, 1989.

Morrison, J., and Herbstein, J. Secondary affective disorder in women with somatization disorder. *Comprehensive Psychiatry* 29:433–440, 1988.

Murphy, G.E. The clinical management of hysteria. *JAMA* 247:2559–2564, 1982.

Myers, J.K.; Weissman, M.M.; Tischler, G.L.; Holzer, C.E., III; Leaf, P.J.; Orvaschel, H.; Anthony, J.C.; Boyd, J.H.; Burke, J.D., Jr.; Kramer, M.; and Stoltzman, R. Six-month prevalence of psychiatric disorders in three communities. *Archives of General Psychiatry* 41:959–967, 1984.

Oken, D. The management of the somatizer. *Psychiatria Fennica* 15:53–62, 1984.

Orenstein, H. Briquet's syndrome in association with depression and panic: A reconceptualization of Briquet's syndrome. *American Journal of Psychiatry* 146:334–338, 1989.

Orenstein, H., and Raskind, M.A. Polycystic ovary disease in two patients with Briquet's disorder. *American Journal of Psychiatry* 140:1202–1204, 1983.

Orenstein, H.; Raskind, M.A.; Wyllie, D.; Raskind, W.H.; and Soules, M.R. Polysymptomatic complaints and Briquet's syndrome in polycystic ovary disease. *American Journal of Psychiatry* 143:768–771, 1986.

Othmer, E., and DeSouza, C. A screening test for somatization disorder (hysteria). *American Journal of Psychiatry* 142:1146–1149, 1985.

Oxman, T.E., and Barrett, J. Depression and hypochondriasis in family practice patients with somatization disorder. *General Hospital Psychiatry* 7:321–329, 1985.

Perley, M.J., and Guze, S.B. Hysteria—The stability and usefulness of clinical criteria. *New England Journal of Medicine* 266:421–426, 1962.

Pittman, R.K., and Moffett, P.S. Somatization disorder (Briquet's syndrome) in a male veteran. *Journal of Nervous and Mental Disease* 169:462–466, 1981.

Purtell, J.J.; Robins, E.; and Cohen, M.E. Observations on clinical aspects of hysteria—A quantitative study of 50 hysteria patients and 156 control subjects. *JAMA* 146:902–909, 1951.

Quality Assurance Project. Treatment outlines for the management of the somatoform disorders. *Australia and New Zealand Journal of Psychiatry* 19:397–407, 1985.

Reich, J.; Tupin, J.P.; and Abramowitz, S.I. Psychiatric diagnosis of chronic pain patients. *American Journal of Psychiatry* 140:1495–1498, 1983.

Reveley, M.A.; Woodruff, R.A., Jr.; Robins, L.N.; Taibleson, M.; Reich, T.; and Helzer, J. Evaluation of a screening interview for Briquet's syndrome (hysteria) by the study of medically ill women. *Archives of General Psychiatry* 34:145–149, 1977.

Ritvo, J.H., and Thompson, T.L., II. A 49-year-old clinic for chronically ill somatizers. *Hospital and Community Psychiatry* 37:631–633, 1986.

Robins, E., and O'Neal, P. Clinical features of hysteria in children, with a note on prognosis. A two to seventeen year follow-up study of 41 patients. *The Nervous Child* 10:246–271, 1953.

Robins, E.; Purtell, J.J.; and Cohen, M.E. "Hysteria" in men. *New England Journal of Medicine* 246:677–685, 1952.

Robins, L.N.; Helzer, J.E.; Weissman, M.M.; Orvaschel, H.; Gruenberg, E.; Burke, J.D.; and Regier, D.A. Lifetime prevalence of specific psychiatric disorders in three sites. *Archives of General Psychiatry* 41:949–958, 1984.

Rounsaville, B.J.; Harding, P.S.; and Weissman, M.M. Single case study—Briquet's syndrome in a man. *Journal of Nervous and Mental Disease* 167:364–367, 1979.

Routh, D.K., and Ernst, A.R. Somatization disorder in relatives of children and adolescents with functional abdominal pain. *Journal of Pediatric Psychology* 9:427–437, 1984.

Saxena, S.; Nepal, M.K.; and Mohan, D. DSM-III axis I diagnoses of Indian psychiatric patients with somatic symptoms. *American Journal of Psychiatry* 145:1023–1024, 1988.

Scallet, A.; Cloninger, C.R.; and Othmer, E. The management of chronic hysteria: A review and double-blind trial of electrosleep and other relaxation methods. *Diseases of the Nervous System* 37:347–353, 1976.

Schoenberg, B., and Senescu, R. Group psychotherapy for patients with chronic multiple somatic complaints. *Journal of Chronic Disease* 19:649–657, 1966.

Schreter, R.K. Treating the untreatables: A group experience with somaticizing borderline patients. *International Journal of Psychiatry in Medicine* 10:205–215, 1980.

Schulberg, H.C., and Burns, B.J. Mental disorders in primary care: Epidemiologic, diagnostic, and treatment research directions. *General Hospital Psychiatry* 10:79–87, 1988.

Schurman, R.A.; Kramer, P.D.; and Mitchell, J.B. The hidden mental health network. *Archives of General Psychiatry* 42:89–94, 1985.

Sheehan, D.V., and Sheehan, K.H. The classification of anxiety and hysterical states. Part II. Toward a more heuristic classification. *Journal of Clinical Psychopharmacology* 6(2):386–393, 1982.

Sigvardsson, S.; Bohman, M.; von Knorring, A.L.; and Cloninger, C.R. Symptom patterns and causes of somatization in men: I. Differentiation of two discrete disorders. *Genetics and Epidemiology* 3:153–169, 1986.

Slavney, P.R., and Teitelbaum, M.L. Patients with medically unexplained symptoms: DSM-III diagnoses and demographic characteristics. *General Hospital Psychiatry* 7:21–25, 1985.

Smith, G.R., Jr. Toward more effective recognition and management of somatization disorder. *Journal of Family Practice* 25:551–552, 1987.

Smith, G.R., Jr., and Brown, F.W. Screening indexes in DSM-III-R somatization disorder. *General Hospital Psychiatry* 12:148–152, 1990.

Smith, G.R., Jr.; Monson, R.A.; and Ray, D.C. Patients with multiple unexplained symptoms. *Archives of Internal Medicine* 146:69–72, 1986*a*.

Smith, G.R., Jr.; Monson, R.A.; and Ray, D.C. Psychiatric consultation in somatization disorder. *New England Journal of Medicine* 314:1407–1413, 1986*b*.

Smith, R.C. A clinical approach to the somatizing patient. *Journal of Family Practice* 21:294–301, 1985.

Smith, R.C. Somatization in primary care. *Clinical Obstetrics and Gynecology* 31(4):902–914, 1988.

Snyder, S., and Pitts, W.M. Characterizing somatization, hypochondriasis, and hysteria in the borderline personality disorder. *Acta Psychiatrica Scandinavica* 73:307–314, 1986.

Spalt, L. Hysteria and antisocial personality. A single disorder? *Journal of Nervous and Mental Disease* 168:456–464, 1980.

Spitzer, R.L.; Williams, J.B.W.; and Gibbon, M. *Structured Clinical Interview for DSM-III-R Personality Disorders*. New York: Biometrics Research Department, New York State Psychiatric Institute, 1988.

Swartz, M.; Hughes, D.; George, L.; Blazer, D.; Landerman, R.; and Bucholz, K. Developing a screening index for community studies of somatization disorder. *Journal of Psychiatric Research* 20:335–343, 1986.

Swartz, M.; Hughes, D.; Blazer, D.; and George, L. Somatization disorder in the community—A study of diagnostic concordance among three diagnostic systems. *Journal of Nervous and Mental Disease* 175:26–33, 1987.

Swartz, M.; Blazer, D.; George, L.; and Landerman, R. Somatization disorder in a community population. *American Journal of Psychiatry* 143:1403–1408, 1988.

Swartz, M.; Landerman, R.; George, L.; Blazer, D.; and Escobar, J. Somatization disorder. In: Robins, L.N., and Regier, D. eds. *Psychiatric Disorders in America*. New York: Free Press, 1990.

Valko, R.J. Group therapy for patients with hysteria (Briquet's disorder). *Diseases of the Nervous System* 37:484–487, 1976.

Veith, I. Four thousand years of hysteria. In: Horowitz, M.J., ed. *Hysterical Personality*. New York: Jason Aronson, 1977. pp. 9–93.

Weissman, M.M.; Myers, J.K.; and Harding, P.S. Psychiatric disorders in a U.S. urban community: 1975–1976. *American Journal of Psychiatry* 135:459–462, 1978.

Weller, R.A.; Weller, E.B.; and Herjanic, B. Adult psychiatric disorders in psychiatrically ill young adolescents. *American Journal of Psychiatry* 140:1585–1588, 1983.

Wells, K.B.; Golding, J.M.; and Burnam, M.A. Psychiatric disorder in a sample of the general population with and without chronic medical conditions. *American Journal of Psychiatry* 145:976–981, 1988.

Westermeyer, J.; Bouafuely, M.; Neider, J.; and Callies, A. Somatization among refugees: An epidemiologic study. *Psychosomatics* 30(1):34–43, 1989.

Woerner, P.I., and Guze, S.B. A family and marital study of hysteria. *British Journal of Psychiatry* 114:161–168, 1968.

Woodruff, R.A., Jr. Hysteria: An evaluation of objective diagnostic criteria by the study of women with chronic medical illnesses. *British Journal of Psychiatry* 114:1115–1119, 1967.

Woodruff, R.A., Jr.; Clayton, P.J.; and Guze, S.B. Hysteria—Studies of diagnosis, outcome, and prevalence. *JAMA* 215:425–428, 1971.

Woodruff, R.A., Jr.; Robins, L.N.; Taibleson, M.; Reich, T.; Schwin, R.; and Frost, N. A computer assisted derivation of a screening interview for hysteria. *Archives of General Psychiatry* 29:450–454, 1973.

Woodruff, R.A., Jr.; Goodwin, D.W.; and Guze, S.B. Hysteria (Briquet's syndrome). In: Roy, A., ed. *Hysteria*. New York: John Wiley & Sons, 1982. pp. 117–129.

Young, S.J.; Alpers, D.H.; Norland, C.C.; and Woodruff, R.A., Jr. Psychiatric illness and the irritable bowel syndrome. *Gastroenterology* 70:162–166, 1976.

Zoccolillo, M.S., and Cloninger, C.R. Parental breakdown associated with somatisation disorder (hysteria). *British Journal of Psychiatry* 147:443–445, 1985.

Zoccolillo, M.S., and Cloninger, C.R. Excess medical care of women with somatization disorder. *Southern Medical Journal* 79:532–535, 1986*a*.

Zoccolillo, M.S., and Cloninger, C.R. Somatization disorder: Psychologic symptoms, social disability, and diagnosis. *Comprehensive Psychiatry* 27:65–73, 1986*b*.

Annotated Bibliography

Each reference in this bibliography is listed only once, even though it may be relevant to several topics.

Children

Ernst, A.R.; Routh, D.K.; and Harper, D.C. Abdominal pain in children and symptoms of somatization disorder. *Journal of Pediatric Psychology* 9:77–86, 1984.

>A study from a multispeciality primary care setting that supports the development of a childhood disorder similar to somatization disorder.

Kriechman, A.M. Siblings with somatoform disorders in childhood and adolescence. *Journal of the American Academy of Child and Adolescent Psychiatry* 26:226–231, 1987.

>A study of the first-degree relatives of 12 children with somatoform disorders demonstrating the high prevalence of somatization disorder in the women and alcoholism and sociopathy in the men.

Livingston, R., and Martin-Cannici, C. Multiple somatic complaints and possible somatization disorder in prepubertal children. *Journal of the American Academy of Child Psychiatry* 24:603–607, 1985.

>A report on five prepubertal children with multiple unexplained complaints.

Morrison, J. Childhood sexual histories of women with somatization disorder. *American Journal of Psychiatry* 146:239–241, 1989.

>A study of 60 female psychiatric patients with somatization disorder and 31 women with primary mood disorders showed that childhood sexual histories were similar for the two groups except that women with somatization were significantly more likely to have been sexually abused as a child (55 percent vs. 16 percent).

Robins, E., and O'Neal, P. Clinical features of hysteria in children, with a note on prognosis. A two to seventeen year follow-up study of 41 patients. *The Nervous Child* 10:246–271, 1953.

An early study of somatization disorder in children demonstrating the reliability of the multisymptomatic form of hysteria.

Routh, D.K., and Ernst, A.R. Somatization disorder in relatives of children and adolescents with functional abdominal pain. *Journal of Pediatric Psychology* 9:427–437, 1984.

A study of 20 children with functional abdominal pain and controls found that 10 of the 20 children had one or more relatives with somatization disorder.

Zoccolillo, M.S., and Cloninger, C.R. Parental breakdown associated with somatization disorder (hysteria). *British Journal of Psychiatry* 147:443–445, 1985.

A study of 30 patients with somatization disorder compared to controls with major depression indicating parenting problems in patients with somatization disorder.

Comorbidity

Katon, W.; Kleinman, A.; and Rosen, G. Depression and somatization: A review. *American Journal of Medicine* 72:127–135, 1982.

A two-part review that thoroughly addresses the relationship between the process of somatization and depression, especially as it relates to primary care.

Lilienfeld, S.O.; Van Valkenburg, C.; Larntz, K.; and Akiskal, H.S. The relationship of histrionic personality disorder to antisocial personality and somatization disorder. *American Journal of Psychiatry* 143:718–722, 1986.

A study demonstrating the association between somatization disorder, antisocial personality disorder, and histrionic personality disorder in somatization disorder patients and their first-degree relatives. The study proposes that somatization disorder may be the female manifestation and antisocial personality the male manifestation of the same underlying disorder, in this case, histrionic personality disorder.

Liskow, B.; Othmer, E.; Penick, E.C.; DeSouza, C.; and Gabrielli, W. Is Briquet's syndrome a heterogeneous disorder? *American Journal of Psychiatry* 143:626–629, 1986.

A study of the comorbidity of 78 psychiatric outpatients diagnosed with somatization disorder, demonstrating the high prevalence of additional diagnoses in the patients.

Conversion

Coryell, W., and House, D. The validity of broadly defined hysteria and DSM-III conversion disorder: Outcome, family history, and mortality. *Journal of Clinical Psychiatry* 45:252–256, 1984.

A followup study of patients with somatization disorder, hysteria but not somatization disorder, and conversion disorder demonstrates that somatization disorder is different from conversion disorder and that somatization disorder has a lower mortality rate than depression.

Farley, J.; Woodruff, R.A., Jr.; and Guze, S.B. The prevalence of hysteria and conversion symptoms. *British Journal of Psychiatry* 114:1121–1125, 1968.

In postpartum women, the prevalence estimates of hysteria were 1–2 percent. Data demonstrate difference of those with somatization disorder from those with conversion disorder.

Folks, D.G.; Ford, C.V.; and Regan, W.M. Conversion symptoms in a general hospital. *Psychosomatics* 25:285–291, 1984.

Analysis of 1,000 consecutive psychiatric consultations that showed a 5-percent prevalence of conversion symptoms. Of those 50 patients with a conversion symptom, 34 percent had somatization disorder.

Ford, C.V., and Folks, D.G. Conversion disorders: An overview. *Psychosomatics* 26:371–378, 1985.

A comprehensive review of conversion disorders with special attention to conversion symptoms. The authors conclude that conversion should be evaluated as a symptom rather that as a syndrome.

Guze, S.; Woodruff, R.A.; and Clayton, P.J. A study of conversion symptoms in psychiatric outpatients. *American Journal of Psychiatry* 128:643–646, 1971.

Another study that supports the hypothesis that somatization disorder and antisocial personality may share a common etiology.

Woodruff, R.A.; Clayton, P.J.; and Guze, S.B. Hysteria: An evaluation of specific diagnostic criteria by the study of randomly selected psychiatric clinic patients. *British Journal of Psychiatry* 115:1243–1248, 1969.

A study of 100 psychiatric outpatients in which conversion was found in patients of various diagnoses. Little overlap was found between somatization disorder and other psychiatric illnesses.

Course

Coryell, W., and Norten, S.G. Briquet's syndrome (somatization disorder) and primary depression: Comparison of background and outcome. *Comprehensive Psychiatry* 22:249–256, 1981.

A followup study of psychiatric patients with somatization disorder compared to primary depression shows that somatization disorder patients have a more chronic course and are less likely to recover.

Guze, S.B. The diagnosis of hysteria: What are we trying to do? *American Journal of Psychiatry* 124:491–498, 1967.

An early review of work toward establishing the validity of somatization disorder with special focus on followup and family studies.

Guze, S.B., and Perley, M.J. Observations on the natural history of hysteria. *American Journal of Psychiatry* 119:960–965, 1963.

A 6- to 8-year followup study of 25 patients with hysteria (somatization disorder) showing that it is a distinct, recognizable multisymptomatic illness with a chronic course. There were few, if any, remissions.

Guze, S.B.; Cloninger, C.R.; Martin, R.L.; and Clayton, P.J. A follow-up and family study of Briquet's syndrome. *British Journal of Psychiatry* 149:17–23, 1986.

A followup study of 36 cases of somatization disorder and 26 probable cases drawn from a population of psychiatric outpatients. Also includes the study of their first-degree relatives. Demonstrates diagnostic consistency over many years. Female first-degree relatives have increased risk for somatization disorder and antisocial personality while male relatives have increased risk for antisocial personality.

Perley, M.J., and Guze, S.B. Hysteria—The stability and usefulness of clinical criteria. *New England Journal of Medicine* 266:421–426, 1962.

Followup study confirmed findings by Cohen et al. that there was diagnostic stability using the criteria in multisymptomatic patients with somatization disorder. Patients meeting specific criteria have a 90-percent probability of meeting the criteria in 6–8 years.

Woodruff, R.A., Jr.; Goodwin, D.W.; and Guze, S.B. Hysteria (Briquet's syndrome). In: Roy, A., ed. *Hysteria.* New York: John Wiley & Sons, 1982. pp. 117–129.

A review of studies about somatization disorder with emphasis on evaluation of the concept of the disorder and its management.

Depression

Bibb, R.C., and Guze, S.B. Hysteria (Briquet's syndrome) in a psychiatric hospital: The significance of secondary depression. *American Journal of Psychiatry* 129:224–228, 1972.

Study of women on a psychiatry inpatient service indicating that 10 percent of the admissions have somatization disorder. Depression, substance abuse, and suicide threats are common in these patients.

Maany, I. Treatment of depression associated with Briquet's syndrome. *American Journal of Psychiatry* 138:373–376, 1981.

Presentation of two cases of somatization disorder complicated by depression.

Morrison, J., and Herbstein, J. Secondary affective disorder in women with somatization disorder. *Comprehensive Psychiatry* 29:433–440, 1988.

Sixty women with somatization disorder were compared with 29 women with either unipolar or bipolar depression. Of the patients with somatization disorder, 54 (90 percent) had a lifetime history of a major depressive episode. The somatization disorder patients generally reported more severe depressive episodes and more psychiatric readmissions.

Orenstein, H. Briquet's syndrome in association with depression and panic: A reconceptualization of Briquet's syndrome. *American Journal of Psychiatry* 146:334–338, 1989.

In a consecutive sample of psychiatric patients, somatization disorder was significantly more common in patients who had both major depression and panic than in patients who had either alone. The author suggests a common etiological diathesis for these disorders.

Oxman, T.E., and Barrett, J. Depression and hypochondriasis in family practice patients with somatization disorder. *General Hospital Psychiatry* 7:321–329, 1985.

Thirteen primary care patients were studied for the presence of hypo-chondriasis and depression. Data suggest the separation of hypochon-driasis from somatization disorder and the need for better definitions of depression in these patients.

Diagnosis

Ford, C.V. The somatizing disorders. *Psychosomatics* 27:327–337, 1986.

An excellent review of all of the somatization disorders. Diagnostic and management considerations are discussed.

Ford, C.V. Somatization. In: Soreff, S.M., and McNeil, G.N., eds. *Handbook of Psychiatric Differential Diagnosis.* Littleton, MA: PSG, 1987. pp. 195–235.

A review of the differential diagnosis of the somatoform disorders with an excellent section on somatization disorder.

Guze, S.B. The validity and significance of the clinical diagnosis of hysteria (Briquet's syndrome). *American Journal of Psychiatry* 132:138–141, 1975.

The author outlines diagnostic validity as essential for progress in psychiatric research. Diagnostic validity includes a clear description, common etiology, uniform course, and increased prevalence in family members. These are then related to hysteria.

Katon, W.; Ries, R.K.; and Kleinman, A. Part II: A prospective DSM-III study of 100 consecutive somatization patients. *Comprehensive Psychiatry* 25:305–314, 1984.

A prospective study of 100 patients from primary care who were referred for psychiatric consultation because of the amount of somatization. A variety of psychiatric diagnoses were found, but only 6 percent met criteria for somatization disorder.

Smith, R.C. A clinical approach to the somatizing patient. *Journal of Family Practice* 21:294–301, 1985.

A review of the diagnosis and management of somatizing patients in primary care.

Swartz, M.; Hughes; D.; Blazer, D.; and George, L. Somatization disorder in the community—A study of diagnostic concordance among three diagnostic systems. *Journal of Nervous and Mental Disease* 175:26–33, 1987.

A study of the diagnostic concordance in a general population survey showing that the various criteria for somatization disorder identify roughly the same people.

Disability

Zoccolillo, M.S., and Cloninger, C.R. Somatization disorder: Psychologic symptoms, social disability, and diagnosis. *Comprehensive Psychiatry* 27:65–73, 1986.

A study of 50 psychiatric outpatients with somatization disorder and controls with major depression. Patients with somatization disorder were greatly disabled in work, social activities, and parenting.

Epidemiology

Cloninger, C.R.; Martin, R.L.; Guze, S.B.; and Clayton, P.J. A prospective follow-up and family study of somatization in men and women. *American Journal of Psychiatry* 143:873–878, 1986.

A prospective followup study of psychiatric outpatients. Prevalence of somatization disorder in psychiatric outpatients was 22 percent. Somatization was very rare in men. Clear familial aggregation in women who met Briquet's syndrome criteria was found.

deGruy, F.; Columbia, L.; and Dickinson, P. Somatization disorder in a family practice. *Journal of Family Practice* 25:45–51, 1987.

A study of somatization disorder in a primary care setting indicating that 5 percent of the patients had somatization disorder. These patients had 50-percent greater health care utilization and lower socioeconomic status.

deGruy, F.; Crider, J.; Hashimi, D.K.; Dickinson, P.; Mullins, H.C.; and Troncale, J. Somatization disorder in a university hospital. *Journal of Family Practice* 25:579–584, 1987.

A study of patients from medical and surgical services of a general hospital demonstrates that 9 percent of these patients had somatization disorder. Fourteen percent of the women had somatization disorder and 3 percent of the men had the diagnosis.

DeSouza, C., and Othmer, E. Somatization disorder and Briquet's syndrome: An assessment of their diagnostic concordance. *Archives of General Psychiatry* 41:334–336, 1984.

A comparison of somatization disorder and Briquet's criteria providing data that they represent similar patients. They show that the prevalence in psychiatric outpatients is 5.7 percent.

Escobar, J.I.; Brunham, A.; Karno, M.; Forsythe, A.; and Golding, J.M. Somatization in the community. *Archives of General Psychiatry* 44:713–718, 1987.

The results from one of the ECA sites which showed that only 0.03 percent of the community sample had somatization disorder. However, 4.4 percent of the sample were somatizers.

Escobar, J.I.; Golding, J.M.; Hough, R.L.; Karno, M.; Burnam, M.A.; and Wells, K.B. Somatization in the community: Relationship to disability and use of services. *American Journal of Public Health* 77:837–840, 1987.

A study that used six unexplained symptoms for women and four for men to define somatizers found that 4.4 percent of the general population meet criteria for trait. The study also found that somatizers had more health care utilization, reported poorer health status, and preferentially used more medical care services compared to other psychiatric patients.

Escobar, J.I.; Rubio-Stipec, M.; Canino, G.; and Karno, M. Somatic symptom index (SSI): A new and abridged somatization construct. *Journal of Nervous and Mental Disease* 177:140–146, 1989.

Data from two community studies demonstrate that an abridged construct of somatization is very prevalent and related to demographic variables.

Kessler, L.G.; Cleary, P.D.; and Burke, J.D., Jr. Psychiatric disorders in primary care. *Archives of General Psychiatry* 42:583–590, 1985.

An epidemiological study of primary care patients indicating that 4 percent have somatization disorder. This is a low rate compared to other primary care studies.

Martin, R.L.; Roberts, W.V.; and Clayton, P.J. Psychiatric status after hysterectomy. *JAMA* 244:350–353, 1980.

A study of 49 patients who had noncancer hysterectomies. The study found that 27 percent of these women had somatization disorder.

Purtell, J.J.; Robins, E.; and Cohen, M.E. Observations on clinical aspects of hysteria—A quantitative study of 50 hysteria patients and 156 control subjects. *JAMA* 146:902–909, 1951.

First modern study of multisymptomatic patients with hysteria. Observed 50 patients at diagnosis and 4 or more months later. Suggested that men do not have hysteria. Prevalence in a general hospital: 2.2 percent. Noted similarity to Briquet's work.

Reich, J.; Tupin, J.P.; and Abramowitz, S.I. Psychiatric diagnosis of chronic pain patients. *American Journal of Psychiatry* 140:1495–1498, 1983.

Twelve percent of chronic pain patients had somatization disorder.

Swartz, M.; Blazer, D.; George, L.; and Landerman, R. Somatization disorder in a community population. *American Journal of Psychiatry* 143:1403–1408, 1988.

A report from a large epidemiology study of the general population indicating the prevalence of somatization disorder is at 0.38 percent.

Swartz, M.; Landerman, R.; George, L.; Blazer, D.; and Escobar, J. Somatization disorder. In: Robins, L.N., and Regier, D. eds. *Psychiatric Disorders in America*. New York: Free Press, 1990.

A thorough presentation of Epidemiology Catchment Area project's findings concerning somatization disorder.

Young, S.J.; Alpers, D.H.; Norland, C.C.; and Woodruff, R.A., Jr. Psychiatric illness and the irritable bowel syndrome. *Gastroenterology* 70:162–166, 1976.

A study of psychiatric diagnoses in patients with irritable bowel syndrome. They found that 17 percent had somatization disorder.

Family

Arkonac, O., and Guze, S.B. A family study of hysteria. *New England Journal of Medicine* 268:239–242, 1963.

A study of 172 first-degree relatives of patients with somatization disorder indicating an increased prevalence of somatization disorder in female relatives and alcoholism and possibly antisocial personality in the men.

Cloninger, C.R., and Guze, S.B. Hysteria and parental psychiatric illness. *Psychological Medicine* 5:27–31, 1975.

A two-generation study of 46 families of convicted women showed that the daughters of sociopathic fathers had a significantly higher prevalence of hysteria than did the daughters of other fathers. The differences were for daughters with hysteria plus sociopathy and for hysteria without sociopathy. The association was of assortative mating between sociopathic men and women with hysteria or sociopathy.

Cloninger, C.R.; Reich, T.; and Guze, S.B. The multifactorial model of disease transmission. III: Familial relationship between sociopathy and hysteria (Briquet's syndrome). *British Journal of Psychiatry* 127:23–32, 1975.

A study that provides further evidence of somatization disorder and antisocial personality clustering in families. This study argues that the two disorders are manifestations of the same process.

Cloninger, C.R.; Martin, R.L.; Guze, S.B.; and Clayton, P.J. A prospective follow-up and family study of somatization in men and women. *American Journal of Psychiatry* 143:873–878, 1986.

A prospective followup study of psychiatric outpatients. Prevalence of somatization disorder in psychiatric outpatients was 22 percent. Somatization was very rare in men. Clear familial aggregation in women who met Briquet's syndrome criteria was found.

Coryell, W. A blind family history study of Briquet's syndrome. *Archives of General Psychiatry* 37:1266–1269, 1980.

A followup chart study of 49 patients with somatization disorder that supports the validity of the syndrome.

Guze, S.B. Studies in hysteria. *Canadian Journal of Psychiatry* 28:434–437, 1983.

An historical and scientific account of somatization disorder as it has evolved, by the researcher primarily responsible for most of the work, Samuel B. Guze, M.D. The account argues for increased prevalence of somatization disorder in female first-degree relatives of somatization disorder patients and of antisocial personality and alcoholism in male relatives.

Guze, S.B.; Cloninger, C.R.; Martin, R.L.; and Clayton, P.J. A follow-up and family study of Briquet's syndrome. *British Journal of Psychiatry* 149:17–23, 1986.

A followup study of 36 cases of somatization disorder and 26 probable cases drawn from a population of psychiatric outpatients. Also includes the study of their first-degree relatives. Demonstrates diagnostic consistency over many years. Female first-degree relatives have increased risk for somatization disorder and antisocial personality while male relatives have increased risk for antisocial personality.

Group Treatment

Corbin, L.; Hanson, R.; Hopp, S.; and Whitley, A. Somatoform disorders—How to reduce overutilization of health care services. *Journal of Psychosocial Nursing* 26:31–34, 1988.

Preliminary report of a group treatment approach for patients who are "overutilizers" of health care; in this case, most had a somatoform disorder. The authors report a reduction in unscheduled visits after the group intervention.

Ford, C.V. Somatizing disorders. In: Roback, H.B., ed. *Helping Patients and Their Families Cope with Medical Problems.* San Francisco: Jossey-Bass, 1984. pp. 39–59.

Treatment of somatization is reviewed with special emphasis on group treatment. The efficiency of group treatment is discussed.

Ford, C.V., and Long, K.D. Group psychotherapy of somatizing patients. *Psychotherapy and Psychosomatics* 28:294–304, 1977.

A review of group treatment with somatizing patients that is applicable to somatization disorder.

Mally, M.A., and Ogston, W.D. Treatment of the "untreatables." *International Journal of Group Psychotherapy* 14:369–374, 1964.

A study describing a group treatment approach for patients seen in a medical setting who somatize.

Schoenberg, B., and Senescu, R. Group psychotherapy for patients with chronic multiple somatic complaints. *Journal of Chronic Diseases* 19:649–657, 1966.

A report of an 18-month analytically oriented group treatment of patients with multiple somatic complaints. At a 5-year followup, their health care utilization was substantially reduced.

Schreter, R.K. Treating the untreatables: A group experience with somaticizing borderline patients. *International Journal of Psychiatry in Medicine* 10:205–215, 1980.

A report of a 2-year group treatment of patients with chronic somatic complaints.

Valko, R.J. Group therapy for patients with hysteria (Briquet's disorder). *Diseases of the Nervous System* 37:484–487, 1976.

A report of a group therapy intervention with somatization disorder patients that reduced their outpatient visits and number of medications.

Health Care Utilization

Smith, G.R., Jr.; Monson, R.A.; and Ray, D.C. Patients with multiple unexplained symptoms. *Archives of Internal Medicine* 146:69–72, 1986.

A series of 41 patients with somatization disorder from a primary care setting were studied. They were found to have nine times the U.S. per capita health care expenditure.

Zoccolillo, M.S., and Cloninger, C.R. Excess medical care of women with somatization disorder. *Southern Medical Journal* 79:532–535, 1986.

A study of 50 patients with somatization disorder indicating their excess health care utilization and surgery.

History

Mai, F.M. Pierre Briquet: 19th century savant with 20th century ideas. *Canadian Journal of Psychiatry* 28:418–421, 1983.

An historical account of what is known of Pierre Briquet, the French physician who first described somatization disorder.

Mai, F.M., and Merskey, H. Briquet's treatise on hysteria: A synopsis and commentary. *Archives of General Psychiatry* 37:1401–1405, 1980.

A synopsis of Paul Briquet's treatise describing 430 cases of hysteria. The treatise clearly noted the polysymptomatic presentation and the fact that men have the disorder.

Merskey, H. Hysteria: The history of an idea. *Canadian Journal of Psychiatry* 28:428–433, 1983.

A review of the history of hysteria.

Management

Abbey, S.E., and Lipowski, N.J. Comprehensive management of persistent somatization: An innovative inpatient program. *Psychotherapy and Psychosomatics* 48:110–115, 1987.

The authors outline an inpatient program designed to interrupt the cycle of somatization and improve the persistent somatizers' level of social and occupational functioning. The approach is multidisciplinary and involves four phases: preadmission consultation and screening, comprehensive assessment, multifactorial treatment, and discharge planning and followup.

Cohen, S.I. Somatoform disorders—Symptoms and psychiatric implications. *Hospital Practice* 21(6):165–198, 1986.

Author reviews the presentation, diagnosis, and management of somatoform disorders.

Kaplan, C.; Lipkin, M., Jr.; and Gordon, G.H. Somatization in primary care: Patients with unexplained and vexing medical complaints. *Journal of General Internal Medicine* 3:177–190, 1988.

A comprehensive review of the process of somatization in primary care.

Kellner, R. *Somatization and Hypochondriasis.* New York: Praeger, 1986.

The author discusses the process of somatization, especially as it relates to hypochondriasis.

Lichstein, P.R. Caring for the patient with multiple somatic complaints. *Southern Medical Journal* 79:310–314, 1986.

An excellent review of management approaches for the primary care patient with somatization.

Lipowski, Z.J. Somatization: The concept and its clinical application. *American Journal of Psychiatry* 145:1358–1368, 1988.

The process and somatization disorder itself are both discussed in this review of the concept, its implications for medicine, and its management.

Lipowski, Z.J. An inpatient programme for persistent somatizers. *Canadian Journal of Psychiatry* 33:275–278, 1988.

A paper describing a successful treatment program for patients who somatize in a general hospital setting.

Monson, R.A., and Smith, G.R., Jr. Current concepts in psychiatry: Somatization disorder in primary care. *New England Journal of Medicine* 308:1464–1465, 1983.

A brief review of somatization disorder as seen in primary care.

Morrison, J.R. Management of Briquet's syndrome (hysteria). *Western Journal of Medicine* 128:482–487, 1978.

A review of various management approaches for the patient with somatization disorder, including working with the family.

Murphy, G.E. The clinical management of hysteria. *JAMA* 247:2559–2564, 1982.

A clinically oriented review of management approaches with very helpful personal suggestions.

Oken, D. The management of the somatizer. *Psychiatria Fennica* 15:53–62, 1984.

A thorough review of the management of various somatizing disorders, especially useful in a primary care setting.

Quality Assurance Project. Treatment outlines for the management of the somatoform disorders. *Australia and New Zealand Journal of Psychiatry* 19:397–407, 1985.

An outline of management recommendations for the somatoform disorders, including somatization disorder.

Quill, T.E. Somatization disorder—One of medicine's blind spots. *JAMA* 254:3075–3079, 1985.

A review of management of somatization disorder in primary care settings.

Ritvo, J.H., and Thompson, T.L., II. A 49-year-old clinic for chronically ill somatizers. *Hospital and Community Psychiatry* 37:631–633, 1986.

Describes a clinic in a general medical setting for patients who somatize.

Smith, G.R., Jr.; Miller, L.M.; and Monson, R.A. Consultation-liaison intervention in somatization disorder. *Hospital and Community Psychiatry* 37:1207–1210, 1986.

A summary of work testing a consultation intervention in somatization disorder. A case report of a successfully managed patient is presented.

Smith, G.R., Jr.; Monson, R.A.; and Ray, D.C. Psychiatric consultation in somatization disorder. *New England Journal of Medicine* 314:1407–1413, 1986.

A randomized, controlled crossover trial of primary care patients with somatization disorder indicating that a psychiatric consultation advocating a specific management approach was cost-effective.

Woodruff, R.A., Jr.; Goodwin, D.W.; and Guze, S.B. Hysteria (Briquet's syndrome). In: Roy, A., ed. *Hysteria.* New York: John Wiley & Sons, 1982. pp. 117–129.

A review of studies about somatization disorder with emphasis on the evaluation of the concept of the disorder and its management.

Mechanisms

Drake, M.E.; Padamadan, H.; and Pakainis, A. EEG frequency analysis in conversion and somatoform disorder. *Clinical Electroencephalography* 19:123–128, 1988.

Preliminary study that showed no difference in spectral EEG analysis between somatization disorder patients and controls. There were differences between somatization disorder patients and patients with conversion disorder.

Gordon, E.; Kraiuhin, C.; Kelly, P.; Meares, R.; and Howson, A. A neurophysiological study of somatization disorder. *Comprehensive Psychiatry* 27:295–301, 1986.

Some evidence for a neuropsychological dysfunction in somatization disorder patients.

Gordon, E.; Kraiuhin, C.; Meares, R.; and Howson, A. Auditory evoked response potentials in somatization disorder. *Journal of Psychiatric Research* 20:237–248, 1986.

Preliminary evidence of an abnormality in cortical function as evidenced by auditory evoked potentials in somatization disorder.

James, L.; Singer, A.; Zurnyski, Y.; Gordon, E.; Kraiuhin, C.; Harris, A.; Howson, A.; and Meares, R. Evoked response potentials and regional cerebral blood flow in somatization disorder. *Psychotherapy and Psychosomatics* 47:190–196, 1987.

A study of 14 somatization disorder patients and 14 controls using auditory evoked potentials and regional cerebral blood flow. They found less mismatched negativity in the somatization disorder patients, which suggests that these patients are less capable of distinguishing between relevant and irrelevant stimuli. Further, the blood flow ratio study showed higher right to left hemisphere flow and possibly a hyperactive right posterior region. Both experiments suggest that somatization disorder patients may attend differently to afferent stimuli.

James, L.; Gordon, E.; Kraiuhin, C.; and Meares, R. Selective attention and auditory event-related potentials in somatization disorder. *Comprehensive Psychiatry* 30:84–89, 1989.

Patients with somatization disorder were shown to be physiologically less able to discriminate background (irrelevant) from target (relevant) stimuli. This finding supports Janet's hypothesis of a neurological basis for hysteria.

Orenstein, H. Briquet's syndrome in association with depression and panic: A reconceptualization of Briquet's syndrome. *American Journal of Psychiatry* 146:334–338, 1989.

In a consecutive sample of psychiatric patients, somatization disorder was significantly more common in patients who had both major depression and panic than in patients who had either alone. The author suggests a common etiological diathesis for these disorders.

Men

Cloninger, C.R.; von Knorring, A.L.; Sigvardsson, S.; and Bohman, M. Symptom patterns and causes of somatization in men: II. Genetic and environmental independence from somatization in women. *Genetics and Epidemiology* 3:171–185, 1986.

A study that provides evidence that men and women who somatize are fundamentally different and that somatization in men and women may have different causes.

Robins, E.; Purtell, J.J.; and Cohen, M.E. "Hysteria" in men. *New England Journal of Medicine* 246:677–685, 1952.

A report of early attempts to find men with somatization disorder. All cases of somatization disorder in this series were found to be attempts to seek compensation.

Smith, G.R., Jr.; Monson, R.A.; and Livingston, R. Somatization disorder in men. *General Hospital Psychiatry* 7:4–8, 1985.

Report of a series of new cases of somatization disorder in men indicating that the diagnosis needs to be considered in men with multiple recurrent unexplained somatic complaints.

Screening

Othmer, E., and DeSouza, C. A screening test for somatization disorder (hysteria). *American Journal of Psychiatry* 142:1146–1149, 1985.

Reports the development of two screening indexes for somatization disorder, one of which was incorporated into DSM-III.

Paisson, N., and Kaij, L. Development of a screening method for probable somatizing syndromes. *Acta Psychiatrica Scandinavica* 72:69–73, 1985.

A study of the process of somatization in 50 primary care patients. Proposes a questionnaire as a screening index.

Reveley, M.A.; Woodruff, R.A., Jr.; Robins, L.N.; Taibleson, M.; Reich, T.; and Helzer, J. Evaluation of a screening interview for Briquet's syndrome (hysteria) by the study of medically ill women. *Archives of General Psychiatry* 34:145–149, 1977.

Reports on a test of a previously described screening interview for somatization disorder in women who were medically ill.

Swartz, M.; Hughes, D.; George, L.; Blazer, D.; Landerman, R.; and Bucholz, K. Developing a screening index for community studies of somatization disorder. *Journal of Psychiatric Research* 20:335–343, 1986.

A study relating the development of an 11-item screening index for somatization disorder. This instrument works very well in the general population.

Woodruff, R.A.; Robins, L.N.; Taibleson, M.; Reich, T.; Schwin, R.; and Frost, N. A computer assisted derivation of a screening interview for hysteria. *Archives of General Psychiatry* 29:450–454, 1973.

Report on the development of a screening interview for somatization disorder.

Substance Abuse

Liskow, B.; Penick, E.C.; Powell, B.J.; Haefele, W.F.; and Campbell, J.L. Inpatients with Briquet's syndrome: Presence of additional psychiatric syndromes and MMPI results. *Comprehensive Psychiatry* 27:461–470, 1986.

A study of 16 patients with somatization disorder and 32 controls demonstrating the presence of comorbid conditions such as alcoholism, substance abuse, antisocial personality, and schizophrenia. The authors also suggest an MMPI screening scale for somatization disorder.

Martin, R.L.; Cloninger, C.R.; and Guze, S.B. The natural history of somatization and substance abuse in women criminals: A six year follow-up. *Comprehensive Psychiatry* 23:528–536, 1982.

A 6–year followup of 66 female felons; 41 percent qualified for a diagnosis of somatization disorder. Shows the association of somatization disorder and antisocial personality and, to a lesser extent, substance abuse.

Index

psychiatric disorders in primary care
settings, 13–14
psychiatric service use, 19
somatization disorder in the general
population, 15–17
work disability, 48
Primary care settings
depression and somatization
disorder comorbidity, 25
mental health care in, 13–14
prevalence in outpatient, 20
Psychiatric clinic settings,
somatization disorder prevalence,
17
Psychiatric comorbidity, 9, 25–26, 58,
59
Psychiatric consultation after positive
screen, 31
Psychiatric service use prevalence, 19
Psychosocial mechanisms, 9–10

Referrals, 42, 52–53, 64
Relaxation therapy, 47

SCID II. *See* Structured Clinical
Interview for DSM-III-R
Personality Disorders
Screening
indices, 29, 31–32
questions, 63
Scripts
becoming patient's main physician,
64
disability request, 64–65
referral, 64
screening and diagnostic questions,
63
Self-perception of somatization
disorder patients, 24, 60
Sexual abuse correlation, 22, 58
Simple phobia treatment, 46
SLE. *See* Systemic lupus
erythematosus

Social phobia treatment, 46
Somatized anxiety, 34–35
Somatized depression, 35
Somatizers, 33–34
Somatoform pain disorder, 37
Stress and relapse correlation, 23
Structured Clinical Interview for
DSM-III-R Personality Disorders,
26
Substance abuse. *See* Alcohol abuse
and dependence; Drug abuse
Swartz et al. screening index, 31, 32
Symptom treatment
anxiety disorders, 46–47
comorbid medical conditions, 47–48
depression, 45–46
work disability, 48
Systemic lupus erythematosus, 38

Treatment considerations
chronic condition management,
41–44
consultation, 51
electrosleep, 50
group treatment, 49–50
joint care, 51
patient/physician relationship
importance, 55–57
referrals, 52–53
symptom treatment, 45–48
See also Diagnostic considerations
Tricyclic antidepressants, 45

Visits to primary care physician
avoiding diagnostic procedures, 44
interval between, 42–43, 55–57
mental health care recommendation,
44, 64
new symptom examination, 43–44
regularly scheduled, 42

Wandering uterus theory, 5–6
Work disability, 48, 64–65